CELL BIOLOGY RESEARCH PROGRESS

OSTEOBLASTS

MORPHOLOGY, FUNCTIONS AND CLINICAL IMPLICATIONS

CELL BIOLOGY RESEARCH PROGRESS

Additional books in this series can be found on Nova's website
under the Series tab.

Additional E-books in this series can be found on Nova's website
under the E-book tab.

MUSCULAR SYSTEM – ANATOMY, FUNCTIONS AND INJURIES

Additional books in this series can be found on Nova's website
under the Series tab.

Additional E-books in this series can be found on Nova's website
under the E-book tab.

CELL BIOLOGY RESEARCH PROGRESS

OSTEOBLASTS

MORPHOLOGY, FUNCTIONS AND CLINICAL IMPLICATIONS

HUGO SCHEURER
EDITOR

NOVA BIOMEDICAL

New York

For permission to use material from this book please contact us:
Telephone 631-231-7269; Fax 631-231-8175
Web Site: http://www.novapublishers.com

Library of Congress Cataloging-in-Publication Data

ISBN: 978-1-62417-806-1

Library of Congress Control Number: 2012955913

Published by Nova Science Publishers, Inc. † New York

Contents

Preface

Osteoblasts are highly specialized mesenchymal cells that are mainly responsible for the formation and maintenance of the skeletal architecture. They produce extracellular matrix proteins and are regulators of matrix mineralization during bone formation and remodeling. In this book, the authors discuss the morphology, functions and clinical implications of osteoblasts. Topics include osteoblasts under mechanical strain; mesenchymal stem cells (MSC) into osteoblasts for bone tissue engineering; osteoblast function and their role in skeletal bone diseases; bone morphogenetic proteins (BMP) and osteoblastogenesis inhibitors; the effect of molecular and biochemical differentiation agents on bone formation; and the evaluation of characteristics of osteoblasts and factors related to osteoblastic differentiation and mineralization.

Chapter 1 - Osteoblasts are key components of the bone multicellular unit and have a seminal role in bone remodeling, an essential function for the maintenance of the structural integrity and metabolic capacity of the skeleton. The coordinated function of skeletal cells is regulated by a number of hormones, growth factors and mechanical stimuli that act via interconnected signaling networks, resulting in the activation of specific transcription factors and in turn, their target genes. Bone cells are responsive to mechanical cues and this is of pivotal importance towards biomechanical strategies for the treatment of osteodegenerative diseases. The present chapter discusses the molecular pathways and players triggered by mechanical stimulation during osteoblastic growth, differentiation and activity in health, and also considers the role of such mechanostimulatory approaches in treating various bone pathophysiologies.

Chapter 2 - Stem cell therapies and tissue engineering have opened up a new era of regenerative medicine, promising the replacement or regeneration of any non-functional or damaged body parts. One of the most exciting approaches is, cell-based bone tissue engineering (BTE), which combines living osteogenic cells with biomaterial scaffolds ex vivo to allow the development of a three-dimensional tissue construct. Mesenchymal stem cells (MSC) that can give rise to osteoblasts are widely used in bone tissue engineering and regenerative therapies. The extracellular matrix (ECM) surrounding the cells play significant role in regulating differentiation and development. An ideal scaffold used for BTE should mimic the beneficial properties of the native tissue ECM for tissue regeneration. ECM based scaffolds are reported to support and enhance the differentiation of MSC into osteoblasts and its maturation. The biomimetic surface coating, that mimic in vivo microenvironment, further improves osteoconductivity of implants and scaffolds and is a key for developing functional tissue for various orthopaedic and bone tissue engineering applications. In this chapter, the authors will review currently available paradigms governing differentiation of MSC into osteoblast for bone tissue engineering and understand the role of extracellular matrices, biomimetic scaffolds and various biomaterials that enhance the osteogenesis for bone tissue engineering.

Chapter 3 - Osteoblasts are highly specialized mesenchymal cells that are responsible for the formation and maintenance of the skeletal architecture. They produce extracellular matrix proteins and are regulators of matrix mineralization during bone formation and remodeling. Osteoblasts regulate the activity of osteoclasts through the secretion of cytokines such as receptor activator of nuclear factor κ-B ligand, macrophage colony stimulating factor and osteoprotegerin. In many pathological conditions, bone formation and remodeling are dysregulated and osteoblasts have a major role in the pathogenesis of these disorders. Abnormalities in the differentiation and functions of osteoblasts occur in several common human diseases such as osteoporosis and osteoarthritis. In late-stage osteoporosis, osteoblasts exhibit decreased proliferation rates and abnormal functions, while in osteoarthritis abnormal behaviors and metabolism are observed. There are also some rare human diseases, such as van Buchem's disease, in which osteoblast activity is increased leading to a high bone mass phenotype. In addition, some solid tumors metastasize to the skeleton as a result of dysregulated osteoblast activity. This chapter will summarize the current knowledge about osteoblast functions and their role in skeletal bone diseases.

Chapter 4 - Bone-forming osteoblasts differentiate from the pluripotent mesenchymal stem cells (MSCs), through a cascade of signalling events that involves modulation of gene expression regulated by several key transcription factors. The first transcription factor and the master regulator of osteoblast differentiation is the Runt-related transcription factor 2 or RUNX2. Its expression in common chondro/osteoprogenitors is controlled by different homeodomain transcription factors and suppressors. RUNX2 not only plays a critical role in the early stages of development, but regulates bone formation beyond this phase. In differentiating osteoblasts, RUNX2 induces the expression of Osterix (OSX/SP7) an osteoblast-specific transcription factor. In genetic experiments, *Osx* inactivation in mice results in perinatal lethality, undifferentiated osteoblasts and complete absence of endochondral and intramembranous bone formation. Once committed, preosteoblasts become functional mainly because of ATF4 transcriptional activity which regulates the synthesis and secretion of type I collagen.

Genetic mutations leading to impaired osteoblastogenesis have been associated with several human diseases. A heterozygous mutation of the human *RUNX2* gene causes Cleidocranial dysplasia (CCD), condition characterized by a delay in fontanelles closure and hypoplasic clavicles. Recently, a single base pair mutation in the *SP7/OSX* gene was associated to a form of non-collagenous osteogenesis imperfecta characterized mainly by facial dysmorphism and frequent bone fractures, whereas a loss-of-function mutation in the *RSK2* gene leads to Coffin-Lowry syndrome, an X-linked condition that displays mental retardation and skeletal abnormalities in the affected males.

This review will discuss the key transcription factors involved in osteoblast differentiation and the molecular mechanism of the genetic diseases caused by mutations in these regulatory genes.

Chapter 5 - Bone morphogenetic proteins (BMPs) were originally discovered as factors that induce ectopic bone formation when implanted into muscle tissue and that also stimulate osteoblast differentiation of various cell types. BMPs are the most thoroughly studied of the bone regeneration molecules and have received FDA approval for applications related to bone regeneration in humans. However the clinical utility of BMPs is limited by difficulties with optimal delivery, an identification the BMPs target cells involved in bone regeneration, and a lack of understanding of the systems that modulate BMP signaling or osteoblast differentiation.

In this chapter, the authors will focus on BMP signaling and it's inhibitors in osteoblastogenesis. In addition the authors will discuss therapeutic prospects of bone related diseases such as osteoporosis and bone tissue engineering of bone by using BMP signaling.

In BMP signaling transduction, the BMP-bound type II receptor phosphorylates the type I receptor. The activated type I receptor, in turn, phosphorylates downstream substrates such as receptor-regulated Smads (R-Smads), including Smad1, Smad5, and Smad8, in addition to mitogen-activated protein kinases (MAPKs) such as Erk, Jnk and p38. Smads play a central role among the downstream signaling effectors of BMP receptors and also plays an important role in osteoblast differentiation.

R-Smads phosphorylated by BMP receptors form heteromeric complexes with Smad4 and directly activate the transcription BMP-responsive genes, which include Id1, Id2 and Id3. Both Osterix (Osx) and Runx2 are master regulators of osteoblast differentiation and are also activated by BMP-Smad signaling.

BMP signaling and BMP-induced osteoblastogenesis, are negatively regulated by various factors including MicroRNAs (miRNAs). BMP antagonists such as Noggin, Chordin, DAN family members, and BMP3 prevent the binding of BMPs to their receptors in the extracellular space. A pseudoreceptor, BAMBI, acts as a dominant-negative receptor for members of the transforming growth factor beta (TGFβ) superfamily on plasma membrane. Repulsive guidance molecule (RGM) b/DRAGON also acts as BMP signal inhibitors on the plasma membrane. Smad6 and Smad7 inhibit the kinase activity of type I receptors by direct interaction in the cytoplasm. Smad ubiquitination regulatory factor 1 (Smurf1), a member of the HECT family of E3 ubiquitin ligases, causes the ubiquitination and degradation of Smad1 and Smad5. Protein phosphatase magnesium-dependent 1A (PPM1A) and Small C-terminal domain phosphatase 1 (SCP1), which have been identified as Smad phosphatases, target unknown substrates thereby suppressing osteoblast differentiation in addition to dephosphorylating phosphorylated Smads. Zinc-finger and RAN-binding domain-containing protein 2 (ZRANB2) bind Smads and inhibit Smad transcriptional activity. Several nuclear factors such as Twist, STAT1, Schnurri3, ZPF521, HES, and p53, interact with Runx2 or Osx thereby suppressing osteoblastogenesis. MicroRNAs (miRNAs) are key post-transcriptional regulators of gene expression. Several miRNAs inhibits osteoblastogenesis to bind to target sequence and negatively regulate gene expression, which are important for osteoblast differentiation.

As just described, numerous inhibitors are involved in osteoblastogenesis. Therefore, a precise understanding and novel methods to remove these inhibitory systems of osteoblastogenesis may shed light on the treatment of bone related diseases or tissue engineering of bone.

Chapter 6 - This review concisely discusses bone regeneration using cell therapy. Harvesting bone for tissue grafting is a current problem encountered by craniofacial and oral surgeons. Therefore regeneration of fractured or diseased bone is the main subject in tissue engineering. Stem cells derived from human adipose tissue (ADSCs) are multipotent cells that are able to differentiate into osteogenic, chondrogenic and adipogenic lineages and are potential sources for bone production under effect on several agents. The most common supplemental compounds inducing differentiation of stem cells to bone cells in vitro are Ascorbic acid (AA), B-Glycerophosphate (BGP), Dexamethasone (Dex), Bone morphogenic protein 2(BMP-2) Collagen I (col I), and Vetronectin. Information is accommodating on the most important effector that interaction with stem cells and induced differentiation of osteoblast. This present review; try to give a comprehensiveoverview on molecular and biochemical effects of osteoprecursor cells inducers.

Chapter 7 - Osteoblasts play a key role in bone formation and it expresses bone-related protein such as bone sialoprotein and osteocalcin. The morphology of osteoblast may change related to the environment. The attachment, proliferation and differentiation depend on the local and systemic condition. There are so many diseases that are related to the function of osteoblasts. It is widely accepted that estrogen deficiency may be the principal cause of postmenopausal osteoporosis, and that the direct effects of estrogen on bone-forming osteoblasts is very important in the progression of the disease.

In this review, the change of the osteoblasts depending on the surrounding environment is describd. Moreover, the change of function and clinical implications will be extensively reviewed.

In: Osteoblasts
Editor: Hugo Scheurer
ISBN: 978-1-62417-806-1

Chapter 1

Osteoblasts under Mechanical Strain

Anastasia Spyropoulou and Efthimia K. Basdra*
Department of Biological Chemistry – Cellular and Molecular Biomechanics Unit, University of Athens Medical School, Athens, Greece

Abstract

Osteoblasts are key components of the bone multicellular unit and have a seminal role in bone remodeling, an essential function for the maintenance of the structural integrity and metabolic capacity of the skeleton. The coordinated function of skeletal cells is regulated by a number of hormones, growth factors and mechanical stimuli that act via interconnected signaling networks, resulting in the activation of specific transcription factors and in turn, their target genes. Bone cells are responsive to mechanical cues and this is of pivotal importance towards biomechanical strategies for the treatment of osteodegenerative diseases. The present chapter discusses the molecular pathways and players triggered by mechanical stimulation during osteoblastic growth, differentiation and activity in health, and also considers the role of such mechanostimulatory approaches in treating various bone pathophysiologies.

Abbreviations

AD	Transactivation domain
ADPKD	Autosomal dominant polycystic kidney disease
Akt	RAC-beta serine/threonine-protein kinase
ALP	Alkaline phosphatase
AP-1	Activator protein-1
ATF4	Activating transcription factor 4
bFGF	Basic fibroblast growth factor

* Corresponding author: Efthimia K. Basdra. Department of Biological Chemistry – Cellular and Molecular Biomechanics Unit, University of Athens Medical School, 75, M. Asias Street, GR-11527 Athens, Greece. E-mail: ebasdra@med.uoa.gr; tegk.84@gmail.com. Phone: +30 210 746 2547; Fax: +30 210 779 1207.

BMP	Bone morphogenic protein
BMSC	Bone marrow stromal cell
Cbfa1	Core-binding factor subunit alpha-1
Cbfb	Core-binding factor subunit b
CCD	Cleidocranial dysplasia
c-Fos	Proto-oncogene c-Fos protein
c-Jun	Proto-oncogene c-Jun protein
Cox	Cyclooxygenase
CREB2	Adenosine monophosphate (cAMP)-response element binding protein 2
CsA	Cyclosporine A
DAG	Diacylglycerol
DDD	Degenerative disc disease
Dlx5	Distal-less homeobox 5 protein or homeobox protein Dlx-5
Egr-1	Early growth response factor 1
ERK	Extracellular signal-regulated kinase
FAK	Focal adhesion kinase
FGF	Fibroblast growth factor
GH	Growth hormone
GTP	Guanosine triphosphate
IGF	Insulin-like growth factor
IL	Interleukin
IP3	Inositol (1,4,5)-trisphosphate
JAK	Janus kinase
JNK	C-Jun N-terminal kinase
LIF	Leukemia inhibitor factor
LIPUS	Low-intensity pulsed ultrasound
M-CSF	Macrophage-colony stimulating factor
MAPK	Mitogen-activated protein kinase
MEK	Dual specificity mitogen-activated protein kinase kinase
MEKK	MAPK kinase kinase
MMSC	Multipotent mesenchymal stromal cell
MSC	Mesenchymal stem cell
Msx-2	Homeobox protein Msx-2
NFAT	Nuclear factor of activated T cells
NF-κB	Nuclear Factor kappaB
NLS	Nuclear localization signal
NMTS	Nuclear matrix targeting signal
NO	Nitric oxide
OPG	Osteoprotegerin
OSE2	Osteoblast specific element 2
Osx	Osterix or transcription factor Sp7
PC	Polycystin
PDGF	Platelet-derived growth factor
PDL	Periodontal ligament
PEMF	Pulsed electromagnetic field

PGE2	Prostaglandin E2
PI3K	Phosphoinositide 3-kinase
PKA	Protein kinase A
PKC	Protein kinase C
PLC	Phospholipase C
PST	Proline/serine/threonine rich domain
PTH	Parathyroid hormone
PYK2	Proline-rich tyrosine kinase 2
QA	Glutamine/alanine rich domain
RANK	Receptor activator for nuclear factor κB
RANKL	Receptor activator for nuclear factor κB ligand
RD	Repression domain
RhoK	Rho kinase
Runx2	Runt-related transcription factor 2
RUNT	Runt homology domain
SMAD	Mothers against decapentaplegic protein
SSC	Skeletal stem cell
STAT	Signal transducers and activators of transcription
TGF-β	Transforming growth factor-beta
TNFR	Tumor necrosis factor receptor
TNF-α	Tumor necrosis factor-alpha
VEGF	Endothelial growth factor
VWRPY	Conserved repression "domain" of runt proteins
Wnt	Wingless-type MMTV integration site family

1. Introduction

1.1. Bone Tissue Cellular Structure

The bone tissue comprises a specialized connective tissue that is composed of the bone matrix and five different types of cells. The bone matrix, which is also referred as minerilised or calcified matrix, constitutes of both organic and inorganic components, whereas the five different types of cells present in bone tissue are the osteoprogenitors, osteoblasts, osteocytes, osteoclasts and lining cells [1].

Osteoprogenitor cells are pluripotent mesenchymal cells, which localise on bone surfaces [1]. They have their origin in mesenchymal stem cells (MSCs), often mentioned as skeletal stem cells (SSCs), bone marrow stromal cells (BMSCs) or multipotent mesenchymal stromal cells (MMSCs) of the bone marrow [2]. Osteoprogenitors are cells that have not received the final signal in order to differentiate into osteoblasts, but when the proper conditions and signals occur, for example contact with the non calcified bone, those cells will commit and undergo the osteoblast differentiation pathway [2].

Osteoblasts, the cells responsible for bone formation, are also aligned in bone tissue surfaces, one next to another. They originate from osteoprogenitor cells localised in the periosteum and endosteum and are responsible for the protein synthesis of the bone matrix as well as its mineralization (also referred as calcification) [1, 2].

Osteocytes, the most numerous cells in the bone tissue, are located in cavities, named lacunae, within the calcified bone matrix. They are inactive osteoblasts that have been entrapped inside the mineralised bone matrix. Nevertheless, osteocytes are not "cut off" since they form networks and have the ability to communicate with each other through osseous tubules, gap-junctions and their long cytoplasmic projections, thereby ensuring the supply of nutrients and regulatory factors in their networks as well as waste disposal [1, 2].

Osteoclasts are large, multinucleate cells that come from blood monocyte merger. They localise in bone resorption lacunae, called Howship's lacunae, and play an important role in bone resorption since they secrete acids, collagenase and other proteolytic enzymes that degrade the bone tissue in areas of bone remodeling [1]. More specifically, osteoclasts adhere to the bone tissue region that is to be reconstructed. The contact surface between osteoclasts and bone tissue is increased due to the presence of multiple folds on their cell membrane. In this region, osteoclasts secrete carbonic, citric and lactic acid which dissolve the hydroxyapatite and lead to collagen release. In the same area, fibroblasts, monocytes and macrophages secrete collagenase and other hydrolytic enzymes causing bone deconstruction and remove organic materials through phagocytosis [1].

Lining cells, which are also known as quiescent osteoblasts or surface osteoblasts, are flattened cells with reduced number of cytoplasmic organelles. Those cells originate from osteoblasts that have ceased to be active but have not been entrapped in the osteoid, the newly formed matrix that has not yet been calcified, like osteocytes. Lining cells cover a large region of bone surfaces, protecting them from the degradative action of osteoclasts [1].

1.2. Osteoblasts

1.2.1. Osteoblast Origin and Life Cycle

Osteoblasts originate from the non-hematopoietic part of the bone marrow. In bone marrow's non-hematopoietic part is mounted a group of fibroblast-like stem cells that have the ability of osteoblastic differentiation. These cells are referred as mesenchymal stem cells (MSCs), skeletal stem cells (SSCs), bone marrow stromal cells (BMSCs) or multipotent mesenchymal stromal cells (MMSCs) [2].

These cells are capable to differentiate into mesoderm-type cells like osteoblasts, adipocytes, chondrocytes, and possibly into non-mesoderm-type cells like neurons and hepatocytes, depending on the signal they receive from their environment [2].

At the first stage of its differentiation towards the cell line of osteo-producing cells process, the mesenchymal stem cell is differentiated into the inducible osteoprogenitor cell, the cell that has not yet received the final signal towards osteoblast differentiation, but under the appropriate conditions and signals, like contact with the non calcified bone, it will undergo this differentiation pathway and become a committed osteoprogenitor [2]. The existence of such inducible osteoprogenitor cells is believed to explain the bone tissue ectopic production in non-skeletal tissues [2].

A diversity of molecules is responsible for the differentiation of MSCs towards inducible osteoprogenitors and the differentiation of those to committed osteo-progenitors. Among them are bone morphogenic proteins (BMPs) [3-5], transforming growth factor-beta (TGF-β), leukemia inhibitor factor (LIF), fibroblast growth factors (FGFs), platelet-derived growth factor (PDGF), as well as transcription factors like runt-related transcription factor 2 (Runx2), homeobox protein Msx-2 (Msx2), and transcription factor Sp7 or osterix (Osx) [6].

The next stage of the osteoblast differentiation pathway is the pre-osteoblast, which is a cell predetermined to become an osteoblast. Pre-osteoblasts are capable of cell division, but this capability decreases as the cells go further in their differentiation. Osteoblasts are incapable to perform cell division. A small percentage of osteoblasts gets trapped in the calcified bone matrix and is converted into osteocytes. It is considered that many osteoblasts remain inactive in the bone surfaces as lining cells, cells able to protect from bone resorption [2].

In order for the committed osteo-progenitors to differentiate into pre-osteoblasts, mature osteoblasts and finally osteocytes molecules like parathyroid hormone (PTH), 1,25-dihydroxyvitamin D or 1,25(OH)2D3, gluco cortico steroids, cytokines, TGF-β, insulin-like growth factors IGF-1 and IGF-2 as well as transcription factors Runx2, Osterix, proto-oncogene c-Fos protein (c-Fos), proto-oncogene c-Jun protein (c-Jun) and distal-less homeobox protein Dlx-5 (Dlx5) are needed [6].

Mature osteoblast life cycle is comprised of multiple stages [7]. During its life cycle, the osteoblast expresses all the necessary genes for the production of bone tissue, but not simultaneously. In the first stage, expression of genes associated with cell proliferation (*runx2*, *osterix*) as well as expression of genes that encode for proteins of the bone matrix (collagen and non collagenous proteins) takes place. In the second stage takes place the expression of genes associated with osteoid maturation whereas in the last stage the expression of genes responsible for bone matrix calcification occurs (production of osteocalcin, bone sialoprotein, alkaline phosphatase and osteopontin among others) [7].

1.2.2. Osteoblast Function

Osteoblasts are capable for a variety of specific functions related to: a) the production of structural components of the bone tissue and b) the production of enzymes and regulatory factors that take part in bone production and resorption [8].

Osteoblastic cells are the responsible cells for the production of the structural proteins of the extracellular matrix. The most important of them is collagen type I, which is the main osteoid component. Another protein that osteoblasts produce is osteocalcin which is a non collagenous protein that is secreted during the calcification phase of the bone with the ability to bind strongly with apatite and calcium. They also produce osteonectin, a glycoprotein that binds sodium, collagen and calcium and plays a pivotal role in calcification initiation. Furthermore, they secrete osteopontin or bone sialoprotein 1 which has the ability to bind firmly to hydroxyapatite. In addition, osteoblasts produce the enzyme alkaline phosphatase (ALP), which is involved in the calcification of the extracellular matrix. This enzyme is located in the plasma membrane of osteoblasts and is associated with the formation of new osseous tissue [8].

Osteoblasts are also responsible for the production of growth factors, cytokines and enzymes, necessary for bone formation and resorption. Growth factors produced by osteoblasts are being deposited and remain bound in the calcified bone tissue matrix. On a later stage, when bone resorption takes place and osteoclasts absorb the osseous tissue, those bound growth factors are released and lead to osteoprogenitor proliferation and differentiation into osteoblasts. Those osteoblasts will form new bone tissue and thus another bone remodeling cycle initiates [8].

1.2.3. Growth Factor and Hormone Effects on Osteoblasts

There are three categories of growth factors that influence the osteoblastic activity as well as the effects of other bone growth regulators. These are:

- Members of the TGF-β family that induce osteoblastic differentiation,
- Insulin growth factors (IGFs) which activate *osterix* gene expression and therefore lead to osteoblast differentiation,
- Bone morphogenic proteins (BMPs) that have an autocrine and paracrine anabolic function in bone tissue which is mediated through specific receptors [9].

However, none of these growth factors is specific for osteoblastic cell maturation. Therefore, skeletal tissue specific mechanisms are necessary, and those mechanisms include osteoblast interactions with circulating hormones (including glucocorticoids, sex steroids, PTH or prostaglandin E2 (PGE2), which on their own have known effects on bone biology) as well as the function of specific intracellular mediators which act upon bone-specific transcription factors [10].

Other growth factors, like the vascular endothelial growth factor (VEGF), the platelet-derived growth factor (PDGF) and the fibroblast growth factors (FGFs), are secreted by vessels surrounding bone tissue and are mainly involved in the process of angiogenesis.

In addition, VEGF has been shown to induce osteoblast differentiation and increase the deposition of minerals in the newly formed bone [11]. The role of PDGF is limited to conditions associated with inflammation and repair while FGFs have been demonstrated to stimulate osteoblast and chondrocyte proliferation but on the other hand, suppress the synthesis of new collagen in the bone matrix [12].

1.3. Runx2 Transcription Factor in Bone Biology

1.3.1. Runx2 in Osteoblast Differentiation

Runt-related transcription factor 2 (Runx2) or core-binding factor subunit alpha-1 (Cbfa1) is an essential osteo-specific transcription factor and a member of the Runt homology family of transcription factors [13]. It comprises a master regulator of osteoblast differentiation since it binds to the promoter regions of all significant osteoblast-specific genes (*osteocalcin*, *type I collagen a3*, *bone sialoprotein*, *alkaline phosphatase*, *osteopontin* and *collagenase III*), controlling their expression [13-15].

More specifically, Runx2 binds to the *cis*-element osteoblast specific element 2 (OSE2) on the promoter of all osteoblast-associated genes [16]. Runx2 is not only necessary for osteoblast differentiation but is also of major importance in the formation of hypertrophic cartilage [10].

It was discovered while investigating the regulation of osteocalcin's expression, which is encoded by a gene expressed only in osteoblasts and in no other cell that produces extracellular matrix components [13, 17-19]. Expression of this transcription factor is necessary and sufficient for the differentiation of mesenchymal cells into osteoblastic cells [20].

All three gene members of the Runt homology family encode proteins that contain a DNA-binding domain and form heterodimers with the transcriptional co-activator core-binding factor b (Cbfb). Cbfb does not bind directly to DNA but allosterically promotes the binding capacity of Runx transcription factors to DNA and increases their half-life, providing stability against proteolytic cleavage through the ubiquitin-proteasome system [16, 21].

1.3.2. Structure of Runx2 Gene

Human Runx2 is encoded by the 220 kb *runx2* gene in chromosome 6p21. The gene contains eight exons and has a similar genomic organization with the other family members, suggesting that the *runx* genes have been conserved during the evolutionary process [22]. Its expression is controlled by two promoters separated by a large intron and exon 1.

The two promoters P1 and P2, produce two main transcripts, type II (starting with the sequence MASNS) and type I (starting with the sequence MRIPV), respectively. Although both isoforms are expressed in osteoblasts and hypertrophic chondrocytes, type I isoform has also been found to be present in non osseous tissues [23].

A third Runx2 isoform, which starts with the sequence MLHSPH, has also been identified, but this isoform is not found in humans [13]. Additionally, it has been reported that alternative splicing generates additional isoforms, which appear to serve distinct cellular functions and which have not yet been determined [16, 23]. The *runx2* gene and Runx2 protein structure is depicted in Figure 1 [16].

The two major Runx2 isoforms (type I and type II), play roles in differentiation of osteoblasts but each one seems to be engaged in different functions in different stages of the differentiation process and of the endochondral and intramembranous bone formation [23].

Type I isoform is shown to be involved in intramembranous bone formation while type II isoform in endochondral bone formation [24].

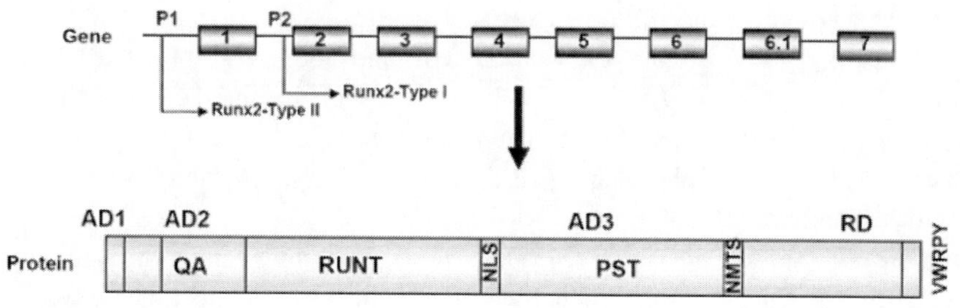

Figure 1. Runx2: gene and protein structure. The *runx2* gene has eight exons and its transcription is modulated by two promoters, P1 and P2. Those promoters lead to production of two transcripts, type II and type I, respectively. Runx2 proteins comprise of AD1-3, transactivation domains; QA, glutamine/alanine rich domain; RUNT, runt homology domain; NLS, nuclear localization signal; PST, proline/serine/threonine rich domain; NMTS, nuclear matrix targeting signal; RD, repression domain; VWRPY, conserved repression "domain" of runt proteins. Reprinted from [16] with permission © 2008 Elsevier.

1.3.3. Runx2 Expression

Runx2 is expressed early during the skeletal development, and is primarily present in developing mesenchymal cells of the regions destined to form bone. In those early stages of embryogenesis Runx2 promotes osteoblast maturation from mesenchymal stem cells [16, 25] while inhibiting it the final stages [25]. During embryogenesis, it can be detected in the spinal chord on day 9.5 and on day 10.5 is strongly expressed in all developing skeletal elements [26]. Runx2 continues to be expressed during post-fetal life, during the procedure of bone formation [16].

Ectopic expression of Runx2 leads to increased expression of osteo-specific genes that encode osteocalcin, alkaline phosphatase, collagenase-3, bone sialoprotein and collagen type Iα1 [13]. Mice with mutation in a *runx2* region are characterised by complete absence of ossification and the intramembranous (mainly through type I) and endochondral (through mainly type II) ossification is completely inhibited due to osteoblast maturation inhibition [16, 27]. Interestingly, stems cells in *runx2* knockout mice did not lose the ability to differentiate into adipocytes and cartilage-forming chondrocytes, a fact that underlines the importance of Runx2 in osteoblastic differentiation. Additionally, heterozygous mice (*runx2* $^{-/+}$) presented skeletal abnormalities that were similar to the ones in the human heritable skeletal disorder cleidocranial dysplasia (CCD) [26]. Even though Runx2 has been shown to be necessary for bone formation, its tissue-specific over-expression in transgenic mice has the opposite results and leads to reduced bone density, bone fractures and osteopenia [16, 28, 29].

Runx2 expression and activity is regulated by various signals like mechanical loading, BMPs, TGFs, PTH and FGF [30]. Given its importance in bone biology, Runx2 expression is strictly regulated through other transcription factors, interactions with DNA or other proteins [20]. Among the transcription factors that regulate Runx2 activity, osteoblast maturation and osteoblast differentiation are Osx, b-catenin, activating transcription factor 4 (ATF4) and Dlx5 [10]. Furthermore, its function is modulated by its interaction with other transcription factors like mothers against decapentaplegic proteins (SMADs) and activator protein-1 (AP-1) [31-33].

Osx is a zinc-finger transcription factor that is expressed only in osteoblasts [34]. Its function is localised downstream of Runx2 [10] and its transcription is shown to be modulated by Runx2 in a positive way [10]. Osx through its interaction with the nuclear factor of activated T cells (NFAT) has been demonstrated to activate the expression of collagen type 1 [35]. On the other hand, p53 decreases *osx* transcription and leads to reduced maturation of osteoblasts [36].

Activation of the wingless-type MMTV integration site family–b catenin (Wnt–b-catenin) signaling pathway results in activation of Runx2. On the other hand when the pathway is inactive osteoblast differentiation from mesenchymal progenitors is blocked, a fact that suggests a role for b-catenin in osteoblast differentiation *in vivo* [37].

ATF4, or cyclic adenosine monophosphate (cAMP)-response-element-binding protein 2 (CREB2), has been shown to interact with Runx2 and modulate *osteocalcin* gene expression [38]. ATF4 plays an important role in osteoblast biology and bone formation since when phosphorylated and thus activated regulates amino acid transportation and is necessary for the synthesis of type I collagen. Inactive ATF4 in mice results in delayed skeletal development and decreased bone mass [39].

Dlx5 homeo-box protein is necessary for normal ossification [40] and is shown to induce Runx2, bone sialoprotein and osteocalcin expression [41]. Osteoblasts with inactive *dlx5* are characterized by decreased proliferation and differentiation as well as reduced Runx2, Osx, osteocalcin and bone sialoprotein expression. Furthermore evidence indicates that Dlx5 modulates bone turnover since it has been demonstrated to directly induce bone formation whereas indirectly bone resorption [42].

Research has revealed an interaction of Runx2 with STAT3b transcription factor. More specifically, it has been shown that growth hormone (GH) which plays an important role in bone biology weakens the transcriptional activity of Runx2 through its physical interaction with STAT3β [30]. More specifically, GH signal leads to extracellular signal-regulated kinase (ERK) activation in osteoblastic cells, an event that suggests that the ERK/mitogen-activated protein kinase (MAPK) signaling pathway mediates GH signaling in osteoblasts. These results suggest that GH confers a regulatory role in osteoblast and/or osteoclast functions. Furthermore, it was shown that GH, that signals through signal transducers and activators of transcription (STATs) / ERKs/MAPKs, increases Runx2 DNA-binding activity in osteoblastic cells lines but attenuates its transcriptional activity. In addition, a direct interaction between Runx2 and STAT3β proteins under GH signal was demonstrated. This interaction was shown to be inhibitory for Runx2 function [30].

To summarize, Runx2 plays a dual role in osteoblast biology. On one hand, it causes osteoblast growth and maturation reduction [43], but on the other hand plays a role in the regulation of expression of genes responsible for osteoblast proliferation and differentiation [44].

2. Bone Remodeling

2.1. Regulation of Bone Remodeling

Bone remodeling is the continuous reconstruction of bone tissue that takes place during our lifetime. This procedure takes place through a catabolic process, the resorption of the old bone by osteoclasts, and an anabolic process, the deposition of new bone by osteoblasts. Bone remodeling is necessary for retaining the structural integrity of the bone and in order for the bone to complete its metabolic functions since it serves as a storage for calcium and phosphorus [45].

The bone remodeling activation phase largely depends on the influence of local factors on the mesenchymal progenitor cells. These cells interact with hematopoietic precursor cells which will form osteoclasts at the resorption phase. Osteoclasts at the end of the resorption process produce a series of signals for bone deposition initiation, which will be carried out by osteoblasts [45].

The reconstruction of the cortical or compact bone begins from groups of osteoclasts which with their function form cavities inside the bone. These cavities become quickly covered with osteoblasts that dispose bone in their surfaces, resulting in their progressive filling with newly formed bone. The reconstruction of the trabecular or cancellous or spongy bone is performed on the surface of the bone. Initially, osteoclasts form a small cavity that osteoblasts fill with new bone. In a young adult, this cycle takes about 200 days to complete. In the cortical bone, the bone remodeling process takes approximately 7 months to complete whereas in the trabecular bone the procedure is shorter, about 3-4 months. In regions of active bone remodeling, bone formation and resorption processes are closely interwoven. Thus, under normal conditions, the amount of newly formed bone is completely equivalent to the amount of bone that has been reabsorpted [46].

1 Quiescent phase: The free surface of the bone remodeling unit is covered by abundant flattened lining cells, which are presently inactive [46].
2 Activation phase: In this phase, an osteoclast stimulator activates pre-osteoclasts and they fuse into large, multinucleate cells in order to form osteoclasts, which are concentrated on the surface of the bone remodeling unit [46].
3 Resorption phase: This phase lasts 3-4 weeks in trabecular bone and 6-10 weeks in cortical bone. During this phase, osteoclasts that have gathered to the free surface progressively absorb the calcified matrix thus emptying the content of the metabolic unit [46].
4 Reversal phase: In this non-fully understood phase, osteoclasts detach and are removed from the bottom of the metabolic unit and in their position osteoblasts make their appearance [46].
5 Formation phase: In this phase, which lasts 2-3 months in cortical and approximately 145 days in trabecular bone, osteoblasts progressive dispose bone, which is normally equal to the amount absorbed in the previous phase [46].

The process of bone remodeling does not require the direct involvement of hormones. However, hormones are necessary to ensure an adequate supply of calcium and phosphorus. On the cell surface of osteoblasts are located receptors for PTH and 1,25-dihydroxyvitamin D, while on osteoclasts no such receptors are present. Therefore, individual osteoclasts do not respond to parathyroid hormone or vitamin D unless they are close to osteoblasts [47, 48].

Research has shown that the GH–IGF-1 axis is of importance in the mechanisms that regulate bone mass quantity and quality. More specifically, GH is suggested to potentially play a role on bone remodeling [30]. However, the mechanisms through which GH acts on osteoblast biology have not been elucidated [49]. GH binds to GH receptors (GHRs) and the signal is transmitted through the Janus kinase 2 (JAK2)/signal transducers and activators of transcription (STATs) towards the nucleus.

2.2. The Role of the RANK / RANKL / OPG System in Bone Remodeling

Although estrogens are the key-hormones controlling the homeostasis of bone, the main modulator of bone remodeling is the receptor activator for nuclear factor κB (RANK) / receptor activator for nuclear factor κB ligand (RANKL) / osteoprotegerin (OPG) system [50]. The common origin of osteoclasts and immune cells is the key to understanding this system and the physiology of bone loss. Osteoclasts and cells of the immune system originate from hematopoietic cells in the bone marrow. More specifically, osteoclasts have their origin in the mononuclear-phagocytic lineage. Macrophage-colony stimulating factor (M-CSF) stimulates the differentiation of cells of the myeloid lineage to pre-osteoclasts. Pre-osteoclasts express in their surface the receptor activator for nuclear factor κB (RANK) which has the ability to bind with its ligand, RANKL. RANKL comprises a tumor necrosis factor (TNF) super-family member that is produced by osteoblasts, stromal cells as well as activated T cells

[4]. Vitamin D, PTH and prostaglandins induce RANKL production on the surface of osteoblastic cells under steady-state conditions. RANK–RANKL binding plays an important role in differentiation towards mature osteoclasts [6, 51].

Osteoblasts derive from the mesenchyme, the network of fetal connective tissue of the mesoderm, from which the connective tissue of the body as well as blood and lymph vessels come from. Adipocytes also originate from the mesenchyme. During normal bone remodeling, cells of the bone marrow-supporting tissue and osteoblasts produce RANKL, which binds to its receptor RANK on osteoclast precursors and causes their differentiation and activation. This occurs through the transcription factor nuclear factor κappa B (NF-κB), which is not only responsible for the activation of osteoclast formation but also for the body's response to inflammation. Both differentiation of osteoclasts and the inflammatory process occur through regulation from interleukin-6 (IL-6). The primary role that cytokines play in bone remodeling is demonstrated by the fact that receptors for the pro-inflammatory cytokines interleukin-1 (IL-1), IL-6 and tumor necrosis factor-alpha (TNF-α) are present both on precursor and mature osteoclasts [52]. Osteoblasts also produce osteoprotegerin (OPG), which is a receptor that blocks RANKL. More specifically, OPG binds through its TNF receptor (TNFR) domains to TNF domains on RANKL [52, 53]. Thus, OPG has the ability to reduce bone resorption and enhance bone formation and therefore it can control bone remodeling process and play an important role in bone homeostasis [52].

2.3. Bone Remodeling Pathophysiology

The health of the bones is maintained by a balanced bone remodeling process that results in the continuous replacement of old bone, which is weakened by microfractures, with new bone. The above procedure comprises of bone resorption by osteoclasts and new bone formation by osteoblasts. Failure in acquisition of peak bone mass or disturbance in bone remodeling may result in pathophysiological bone conditions. Abnormalities in bone remodeling usually result in skeletal disorders such as osteoporosis, Paget's disease, orthopedic disorders and osteopetrosis among others [45].

3. Mechanotransduction

3.1. Bone Remodeling and Mechanotransduction

Bone remodeling is a biological process that results in changes in external and internal bone structure and is largely dependant on the mechanical environment of the bone. Osteoblast and osteoclast functions often compete under specific conditions like the nature of mechanical stimulus applied and metabolic or nutritional stress (Figure 2) [10].

The initial bone response after generation of signals due to local mechanical stress is mediated through bone resorption [54]. However, it has been shown that constant repetitive application of load that causes high stress values as well as the high rates and the unusual distribution of pressure, stimulate osteogenic responses and maintain a high bone mass. On the other hand, application of static pressure as well as slow pressure rotation and application of "predictable" pressure, allow bone loss and low bone mass [55-58]. Additionally, it has been observed an improvement in the bone structure and strength after long periods of mechanical loading when this is interrupted by short pauses [59].

In general the following apply for the bone remodeling process after mechanostimulation: It is promoted by dynamic rather than static mechanical loading. A short-term mechanical stimulation is sufficient to initiate an adaptive response and application of mechanical forces for a short period leads to increased bone formation [60, 61]. Prolongation of this stimulation has a negative effect on further bone adjustment. Furthermore, repetitive mechanical loading leads to a reduction of the response of bone cells due to signaling prediction [58]. The application of these rules is demonstrated in the effects of space microgravity, osteoporosis or paralysis on bone tissues, where bone loss is observed [59, 62], as well as in the effects of tennis at a professional level on bone tissues, where bone growth is observed [63].

The changes in mechanical tension, repair of microfractures and maintenance of the bone remodeling cycle cause cellular responses that are locally modulated by cytokines, growth factors and other molecules. More specifically, interleukin 1β (IL-1β), TNF-α, PGE2 [62, 64], IL-6, IL-8, RANKL, OPG [63, 65-67], IGF, TGFβ-1 and FGF [68-71] have been shown to be induced after application of mechanical stretching. Furthermore, osteoblasts that receive mechanical stimuli exhibit increased expression at the mRNA level of molecules like osteopontin, osteocalcin, PDGF and collagen types I and III [72, 73].

The mechanisms behind mechanotransduction have not been fully elucidated. Mechanical stimulation has been demonstrated to promote DNA synthesis in human osteoblast-like cells potentially through a direct mechanism and not through an autocrine one [74].

The sensor molecules that receive mechanical stimulation should be in close proximity with the plasma membrane so that they receive the mechanical signal and transmit it to the interior of the cell. A number of molecules have been considered to function as mechano-sensors. More specifically, after application of mechanical stimuli, sensitivity and amount of open cation channels [75], gap junctional communication between osteoblasts as well as production of integrins have been found to be elevated [76, 77]. Since deregulation in actin cytoskeleton abrogates the effects of mechanical signaling, the integrin network has been considered as the more probable means of mechanical signal transduction and integrins as candidate mechanoreceptors [78]. However, a group of researchers argue that cytoskeletal components involved in mechanotransduction are specific for different types of stress or responses under investigation [79].

Integrins are transmembrane receptors that connect the extracellular matrix to the cytoskeleton [80]. Important event in signaling through integrins is the focal adhesions and actin stress fibers development [80] mainly with the help of Rho family of Ras-related guanosine triphosphate-binding GTPase proteins [80]. When a signal occurs, integrins form complexes along with cytoskeletal molecules [80]. Members of the Rho family of Ras-related GTPases take part in the formation of those structures [80]. Besides their aforementioned role, Rho family members have the ability to induce multiple kinase cascades and particularly mitogen-activated protein kinase (MAPK) cascades [81]. Rho and other Ras-related GTPases have been shown to play a role in osteoblast response against mechanical forces [82].

MAPK cascades comprise the vessel that carries the extracellular signal in the nucleus and changes gene expression. As far as mechanical signals are concerned, extracellular signal-regulated kinases (ERKs) and c-Jun N-terminal kinases (JNKs) seem to play crucial roles [83-85]. More specifically, ERK signaling has been shown to be involved in altering the expression of osteblast-specific genes after the application of mechanical forces [86, 87]. ERKs and JNKs transmit the signal to transcription factors that alter gene expression, like Jun and Fos family members [88]. c-Jun and Fos family members interact to form activator protein-1 (AP-1) transcription factor, which has been shown to be of major importance in osteoblast differentiation [89-91].

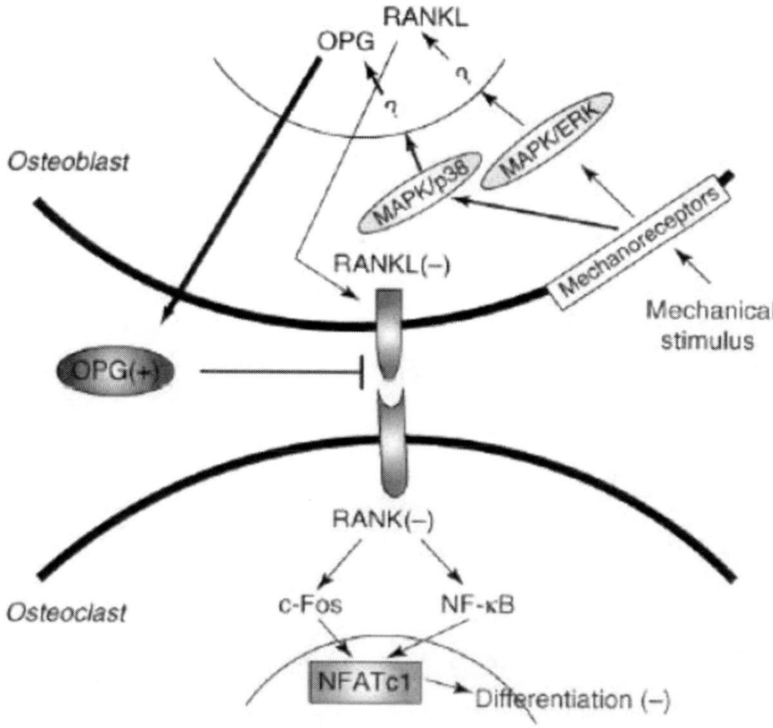

Figure 2. Osteoblast and osteoclast interaction during bone remodeling that occurs after mechanical stimulation that leads to bone formation. When the mechanical stimuli is applied on osteoblasts it leads to elevated OPG production and reduced RANKL expression, and thus RANKL–RANK interaction is interrupted and osteoclast differentiation abrogated. p38 MAPK modulates OPG induction and ERK mediates the activation of transcription factors responsible for RANKL expression. Osteoclastogenesis is regulated by RANK, which activates c-Fos and NF-κB, which in turn lead to NFATc1 activation. OPG, osteoprotegerin; RANK, receptor activator of nuclear factor κB; RANKL, receptor activator of nuclear factor κB ligand; MAPK, mitogen activated protein kinase; ERK, extracellular signal-regulated kinase; NF-κB, nuclear factor κappa B; NFATc1, nuclear factor of activated T-cells, cytoplasmic 1. Reprinted from [10] with permission © 2009 Elsevier.

ERKs have been shown to play a prominent role in osteoblast growth and differentiation [92-94] and their activation has been demonstrated to bear diverse effects on osteoblast cell survival, proliferation, and differentiation [94-97]. In human osteoblast and osteoblast-like cells, ERKs have been shown to be induced by agents that influence bone biology, like growth factors, estrogen, and fluoride [95] but the role of the pathway remains elusive. ERK/JNK signaling pathways have been shown to lead to increased production of Fos and Jun molecules and activate them through phosphorylation, thus altering AP-1 activity [98].

Time, duration and strength of JNK/ERK activation might also be of importance in gene expression [99].

AP-1 transcription factor is important in osteoblast differentiation as it is demonstrated to modulate the expression of genes that encode for collagen type I, osteocalcin, osteopontin and osteonectin [90]. This transcription factor plays an important role in early response after external stimuli [100]. Its components, Fos and Jun family members, are encoded by immediate-early genes that comprise targets of MAPK signaling pathways as mentioned above [98].

In osteoblastic cells, mechanical loading conditions seem to determine the composition of the AP-1 complex and therefore regulate gene transcription differently according the extracellular signal applied [99].

Further research demonstrates that application of continuous mechanical force in human osteoblast-like cells, the human periodontal ligament cells (PDL cells), led into increased production of AP-1 components, c-Fos and c-Jun through activation of MAPK cascades. More specifically, continuous application of mechanical forces results in deregulation in Rab and Rho GTPases activity in osteoblast-like cells [82]. Moreover, continuous application of mechanical stimuli leads to immediate overproduction of c-Fos in osteoblast like cells [101], something that has also been shown in osteoblasts after reception of mechanical signals [102-104]. On the other hand, data about c-Jun after mechanical stimulation is not conclusive. According to Kletsas et al., human osteoblast-like cells after mechanical force application over-express c-Jun [101] whereas others have opposing results [105] probably because of different stress type applied and different cell system used.

When researchers of the same group administrated p38 MAPK, dual specificity mitogen-activated protein kinase kinase (MEK) and Rho kinase (RhoK) inhibitors, the aforementioned results were partially or completely suppressed. Therefore, AP-1 is an important downstream molecule in osteoblast-like cells after continuous mechanical stimulation and its expression is regulated through p38 MAPK, MEK and RhoK pathways [101]. More specifically, the usage of MEK, p38 MAPK and RhoK inhibitors resulted in suppressed c-Fos expression, in different efficacies, in osteoblast-like cells under application of mechanical forces [101] something that is in accordance with existing literature. Accordingly, abrogation of c-Jun expression was observed when those inhibitors were applied in osteoblast-like cells that received the same type of mechanical stimuli [101]. In both cases, MEK and p38 MAPK inhibitors partially suppressed c-Fos and c-Jun expression whereas RhoK inhibitors led to complete suppression [101]. Therefore, it is suggested that RhoK functions upstream of MAPKs in signaling cascades triggered after continuous mechanical stimulation of osteoblast-like cells [101].

In addition, in the same study, the principal modulator of AP-1 activity, c-Jun, was found hyperphosphorylated and therefore its activity was enhanced [101] and this result is in accordance with the previously observed enhanced AP-1 binding activity in human osteoblast-like cells under the same conditions [106]. The usage of p38 MAPK, MEK and RhoK inhibitors downregulated the c-Jun phosphorylation of resting cells as well as reduced the hyperphosphorylation in osteoblast cells that had undergone mechanostimulation, an event that indicates the overlap between signaling pathways in mechanotransduction [101].

According to researchers, application of short-term mechanical forces seems to activate both JNK2 and ERK2, and molecules downstream of those kinases, like c-Jun, alter the expression pattern of genes responsible for osteoblastic phenotypes [106]. More specifically, application of short-term continuous mechanical stimuli of physiological intensity in osteoblast-like cells has been shown to activate JNK and ERK members and lead to increased AP-1 DNA-binding activity on the human *L/B/K ALP* gene [106]. The above result suggests that this kind of mechanical stimulation leads to osteoblast differentiation since increased ALP expression is associated with the onset of the osteoblast phenotype and the formation of new bone [107]. Furthermore evidence supports this suggestion since osteoblast-like cells after mechanical stimulation were characterized by increased type 1 collagen synthesis [108] and increased expression of osteocalcin and those two molecules also comprise determinants of the early osteoblastic differentiation.

Signals of mechanical nature induce in osteoblasts and osteocytes the production and secretion of hormones and growth factors, which modulate osteoblast differentiation and proliferation [10]. More specifically, the effects of hormones and growth factors on osteocytes, the cells that receive mechanical stimuli, result in osteoblast maturation after the application of mechanical force. Such mechanical stimuli can include flow of fluids, strain of the substrate, membrane deformation or stimulation of integrins, vibration, altered gravity forces and compressive loading [10].

PGE2 production is induced in osteoblast-like cells after mechanical stimulation [109]. PGE2 has been shown to be produced in osteoblasts after physiological stress, growth factors, hormones, trauma or inflammatory cytokines and its production leads to cAMP-dependent IGF-1 induction in osteoblasts [10]. IGF-1 and IGF-2, in turn, have been shown to induce Osx expression in osteoblasts [110], induce osteoblast function *in vitro* as well as lead to bone mass increase *in vivo* [111]. The PGE2 effects *in vivo* have also been linked to an elevated Runx2 expression [112]. Downstream of PGE2, TGF-β expression, which has proliferative and ECM production effects in bone [113], has been found increased in human osteoblast-like cells. This evidence accompanied by the fact that TGF-β receptor 1 (TGF-βR1) comprises a Runx2 target in osteoblasts [114] provides an explanation on the fact that Runx2 knockout mice are characterized by defective formation of extracellular matrix due to decreased number of mature osteoblasts [27].

Production of nitric oxide (NO) is another response to mechanical stimuli. The production of NO has been demonstrated in osteoblasts that received mechanical signals. NO interacts with the MEK/ERK cascade since it binds to a regulatory site on Ras and might lead to cell proliferation and ECM production [115]. In a later stage, Cox1, Cox2 as well as ERK1 and ERK2 are activated and result in bone matrix component production [116].

Furthermore, mechanical stimuli result in VEGF-, BMP-2- and BMP-4-dependent and PGE2-independent IGF-1 upregulation [117]. IGF-1 activation results in signal transmission through phosphoinositide 3-kinase (PI3K)– RAC-beta serine/threonine-protein kinase (Akt), MAPKs and SMAD pathways [118]. BMPs function in an anabolic way in osteoblastic cells [118] and signaling after induction by BMP-2 has been shown to promote the expression of *runx2*, *osx* and *dlx5* genes [119].

Signals of mechanical nature also promote the expression of genes that encode for c-Fos, early growth response factor 1 (Egr-1) and basic fibroblast growth factor (bFGF). In addition they have been demonstrated to promote cell growth in MC3T3-E1 osteoblasts [57].

The nature and characteristics of mechanical loading determine whether bone or cartilage formation will take place [120]. When high frequency and low intensity is applied in bone cells *in vitro*, it leads to enhanced ECM disposition and thus bone formation is induced [121].

On the other hand, mechanical loading of high intensity on osteoblastic cells promotes the expression of BMP extracellular antagonists and therefore results in inhibition of osteoblast development [122]. In addition, the application of continuous mechanical forces on osteoblastic cells *in vitro* activates inflammatory cytokines and their receptors production [123]. More specifically, interleukin (IL)-1b production has been shown to be enhanced under such mechanical stimuli, and its production is associated with RANK–RANKL signaling pathway activation and thus bone resorption [124].

Stimuli from short periods of fluid flow or cyclic substrate tension at physiological intensity levels result in osteoblast proliferation and survival [125]. Mechanical signals of physiological intensity levels are associated with survival of human osteoblasts and several studies suggest that pro-survival proteins promote the production of survival factors like IGF-1 or IGF-2 and activate estrogen receptor [126]. It has also been shown that gravitational force retains the survival of osteoblasts. When gravitational force is not applied, osteoblasts are led to apoptosis through reduced DNA binding of a transcription factor that is associated with survival and thus failure of normal mitochondrial activity [53]. On the other hand, when mechanical signals are not present *in vivo*, osteoblasts are led to apoptosis and osteoporosis occurs [120]. The application of excessive mechanical force leads to cell detachment from its surface [127] and results in anoikis, a form of programmed cell death *in vitro* [128]. The complex cross-talk between signaling pathways that take part in mechanotransduction is depicted in Figure 3. Recently, another complex of molecules seems to be implicated in the mechanotransduction of bone cells. Polycystins and more specifically polycystin 1 (PC1), a transmembrane receptor-like protein, and polycystin 2 (PC2), a calcium channel, in co-operation with primary cilia, have been demonstrated to form complexes that localise in specific tissues and cell types, including osteoblasts and osteocytes [129].

Furthermore, absence of PC1 in knockout mice led to abrogated osteoblast differentiation and thus abnormal bone development and osteopenia [129]. Therefore, the polycystins/primary cilia complex may be the missing link in the first steps of mechanotransduction after application of mechanical stimuli.

3.2. Runx2 in Mechanotransduction

The importance of Runx2 transcription factor in osteoblast differentiation and maturation has been studied during the application of mechanical force in osteoblast-like cells and it has been demonstrated that mechanical signals target Runx2 in human osteoblast-like cells [130].

More specifically, application of continuous mechanical loading of low intensity in human osteoblast-like cells of the periodontal ligament (PDL) leads to a direct increase of Runx2 expression and DNA-binding capacity. The signal induction starts from the plasma membrane and more specifically from integrins, which are the proteins that initiate the signal.

This signal, as it has been demonstrated, travels in the cytoplasm through the MAPK signaling cascade and targets Runx2 both at gene and protein levels [130]. More specifically, a signal of mechanical nature results in increased Runx2 expression at both mRNA and protein levels and enhanced Runx2 DNA-binding activity. ERK1 and ERK2 are phosphorylated and thus activated in a time-dependent and parallel manner with the increase in DNA-binding capacity of Runx2. The phosphorylated ERK1 and ERK2 have been shown to interact, phosphorylate and activate Runx2 *in vivo*, which in turn induces osteoblastic differentiation (Figure 4) [16, 130]. These results are in concert with literature that indicates the role of MAPK signaling in osteoblast differentiation [94, 95, 131].

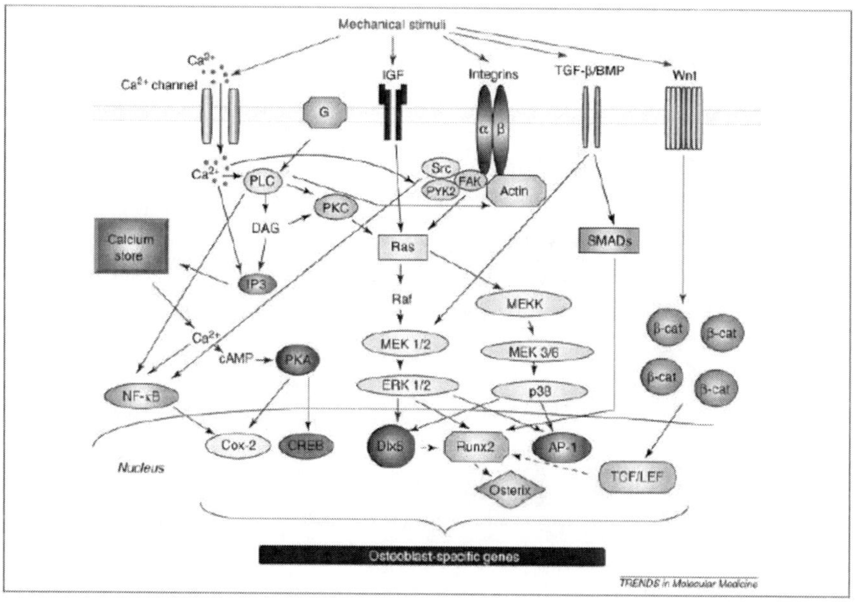

Figure 3. Cross-talk between signaling pathways after application of mechanical stimuli. The signal enters the cell through Ca^{2+} channels, integrins, G-proteins, IGF and TGF-β and/or BMP receptors resulting in activation of signaling pathways like those of MAPKs and SMADs. Those events result in activation of AP-1 and Runx2 transcription factors activation. Activation of the PLC–PKA pathway results in NF-κB, Cox-2 and CREB induction. AP-1, activator protein-1; b-cat, b-catenin; DAG, diacylglycerol; FAK, focal adhesion kinase; G, G-protein; IP3, inositol (1,4,5)-trisphosphate; MEKK, MAPK kinase kinase; PKA, protein kinase A; PKC, protein kinase C; PLC, phospholipase C; PYK2, proline-rich tyrosine kinase 2. Reprinted from [10] with permission © 2009 Elsevier.

Runx2 is known to control its own expression through an autoregulatory mechanism [132]. More specifically, activated by mechanical stimuli ERKs phosphorylate and activate Runx2 molecules that already exist. Those molecules bind to Runx2 promoter and promote Runx2 expression [130]. Furthermore, Runx2 promoter has been found to enclose a canonical AP-1 binding site indicating that AP-1 may play a role in modulating Runx2 expression. In addition, AP-1 and Runx2 proteins have been found to interact and regulate collagenase-3 expression [133].

3.3. Nuclear Factor Kappa B (NF-κB) Transcription Factor in Mechanotransduction

As mentioned previously, the transcription factor NF-κB is associated with the inflammation process [67, 134] but also plays a crucial role in osteoclast formation and bone resorption [30]. NF-κB, which is activated either through the RANK–RANKL system or potentially through integrins that transmit signals of mechanical nature to src-kinases [135], is induced during bone remodeling and stimulates osteoclast formation. Besides all its aforementioned functions, NF-κB probably also stimulates osteoblast differentiation after mechanical stimulation. So far there is only evidence that NF-κB is activated and translocated in the nucleus of osteoblast cells after mechanical stimulus [62, 136] and it is suggested that it may be implicated in the transcriptional activation of osteoblast-specific genes.

3.4. Polycystins in Mechanotransduction

As already mentioned, the initial steps of mechanotransduction remain elusive. Polycystins in co-ordination with primary cilia have been suggested as potential mechanosensor molecules in osteoblasts under mechanical stimulation [129]. PC1 is a large transmembrane protein whose role was investigated in studies on autosomal dominant polycystic kidney disease (ADPKD). Those studies revealed that the N-terminal part of PC1 may function as the mechanical signal "receiver" [137]. Through its C-terminal part PC1 forms a complex with PC2 and together co-localise at the primary cilia, and potentially function there as molecules capable to receive signals of mechanical nature [138]. In addition, it was shown that PC1 regulates the function of Ca^{2+} channels through activation of G-protein signaling pathways [138]. The transduction of the signal takes place through the calcineurin/NFAT axis and leads to the appropriate cell responses [137].

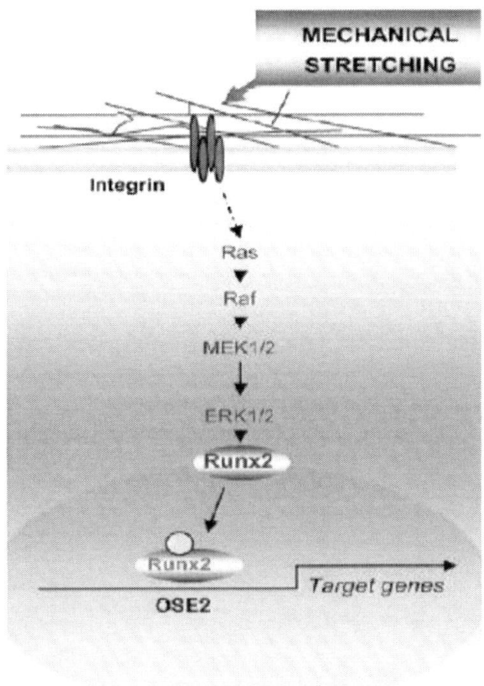

Figure 4. Runx2 activation pathway after mechanical stimulation. Signals of mechanical nature enter the cell potentially through integrins and activate the Ras–ERK1/2 MAPK signaling pathway. Activation of the pathway leads to Runx2 phosphorylation and enhances its transcriptional activity. ECM, extracellular matrix; ERK1/2, extracellular signal-regulated kinase; MEK1/2, ERK1/2 upstream activating kinase; OSE2, osteoblast-specific cis-acting element 2. Reprinted from [16] with permission © 2008 Elsevier.

More specifically, the participation of the NFAT pathway was established by experiments that showed NFATc1 activation after half to one hour of mechanical loading in osteoblast-like cells. In concert with these results, it was shown that administration of cyclosporine A (CsA), a specific inhibitor of the calcineurin/NFAT pathway, to the same system, blocked the decrease of the inactive (phosphorylated) NFATc1 (pNFATc1) form [137]. The same effect was observed when the osteoblast-like cells were administrated with an antibody against the N-terminal part of PC1 prior to mechanical loading. In this case a decrease in the expression of *runx2*, which comprises an NFATc1 target, was also detected [137]. These data suggest that PC1 acts as mechanosensing molecule that modulates osteoblastic gene expression and hence bone-cell differentiation through the calcineurin/NFAT signalling cascade.

3.5. Model Systems for the Study of Mechanotransduction in Osteoblasts

In order to study the role and function of mechanical stimuli in osteoblasts, researchers have used osteoblast-like cells *in vitro* that are acquired either from healthy tissue (human PDL or mouse MC3T3-E1 calvaria cells) or from osteosarcomas (MG-63, SaOs cells). Mechanical signals are transmitted with the help of fluid flow, four-point bending and substrate stretch, gravity force, vibration, magnetic bead twisting, atomic force or shockwaves [139]. The mechanical response of osteoblastic cells has been found to differ depending on the type, duration and level of stress [10].

The system of periodontal ligament (PDL) cells is a helpful model for the study of mechanotransduction signaling in osteoblasts [140]. PDL cells are undifferentiated mesenchymal fibroblasts [141] that bear all the characterized properties of osteoblasts. Those cells are accustomed to mechanical force application, either this is under physiological conditions or under orthodontic treatments. PDL cells under the appropriate conditions and signals can differentiate into more specialized cells in order to assist in the regeneration and repair of the periodontal ligament as well as in the surrounding hard tissue remodeling process [142].

3.6. The Role of Mechanotransduction in Bone Disease

As mentioned before, deregulated bone remodeling is the main cause of a number of bone diseases. Causes of this deregulation could be genetic alterations. For example, *runx2* gene mutation leads to development of the human heritable skeletal disorder cleidocranial dysplasia (CCD) [143, 144]. In addition, Runx2 regulates the expression of genes that are of importance for cancer cell metastasis in bone. Among them are those that encode for matrix metalloproteinases (MMPs) MMP-9 and MMP-13 as well as those that encode for osteopontin and bone sialoprotein [145]. Therefore *runx2* mutation may be responsible for cancer metastasis to bone tissues. Another cause of deregulated bone remodeling is abnormal mechanotransduction. Examples are the development of conditions like ankylosing spondylitis, carpal tunnel syndrome, chronic back pain and disc degeneration. Furthermore, a characteristic example of deregulated mechanotransduction is osteoporosis, which is characterized by enhanced bone resorption and reduced bone formation. Osteoporosis may have its origin in disease, dietary or hormonal deregulation or reduced mechanical stimulation due to long periods of immobility like space travel [53].

3.7. Mechanical Stimulation as a Therapeutic Strategy against Bone Disease

The ultimate goal of theurapeutic strategies against bone diseases is the achievement of increased bone density. Enhanced bone density however is translated into increased bone formation and reduced bone resorption. In order to achieve this, doctors have mostly made use of pharmaceutical treatments like anabolic treatments or treatments with anti-resorptive agents [10].

Mechanical stimulation has been shown to confer the ability to promote bone formation and inhibit bone resorption and thus could be of importance in designing new therapies for bone diseases. Recently, it has been shown that low intensity mechanical signals activate bone remodeling procedures that enhance bone density and ultimately have regenerating effects on bone tissues [146]. In addition, research data have demonstrated that application of mechanical force on PDL and osteoblast cell lines enhanced OPG expression [147, 148] which in turn, led in blockade of the RANK–RANKL interaction and therefore reduced osteoclastogenesis. In addition, mechanical stimulation *in vitro* activated cyclooxygenase (Cox) enzymes and prostaglandins which led in reduced RANKL production and thus abrogated bone resorption [125, 149]. Mechanical stimuli have also been shown to induce the Wnt–b-catenin pathway on osteoblasts and therefore promote osteoblast differentiation and bone formation [150].

Taking into consideration the aforementioned and other results, researchers have turned to mechanical force application in order to treat bone diseases. More specifically, strengthening exercises in osteoporotic patients has been demonstrated to lead to an increase in bone mineral content [151] and physical exercise has been shown to arrest post-menopausal and age-related reduction of bone minerals in the ECM [152]. In addition, the presence and maintenance of a functional mechanical environment seems to be of importance in degenerative disc disease (DDD) and other skeletal deregulations therapy [153]. Mechanical signals in osteoblasts have also been shown to be of assistance in treatment of bone fractures [154]. In this case, ratio [155], form [154] and intensity of loading as well as fracture size [156], are very important in fracture treatment. Moreover, it has been shown that other forms of mechanical stimuli like low-level vibrations at an intensity that cannot harm the bone, comprise a potent preventive mechanism against osteoporosis [157]. Low-intensity pulsed ultrasound (LIPUS) has been suggested to be important in fractures caused by pathological and/or traumatic causes since it has the capability to promote osteoblast differentiation and thus bone formation [158]. Last but not least, extremely low-frequency pulsed electromagnetic field (PEMF) has been shown to induce proliferation and maturation of osteoblasts [159].

The above results indicate that biomechanical treatment may be successful in treating bone degenerative diseases like osteoporosis without the undesirable effects of pharmacological substances administration [146]. Application of mechanostimulation has already a variety of applications in dentistry, orthopedics, the craniofacial development and treatment of fractures.

Conclusion

Bone remodeling is a process necessary for the maintenance of proper structure and metabolic functions of the bone. Dysfunctions in this process can lead to diseases such as osteoporosis, hyperparathyroidism, hyperthyroidism, disease Paget, and osteopetrosis among others. Therefore, the study of the molecular mechanisms behind this process is of paramount importance. In addition, significant effort has been made towards the investigation of the signal transduction mechanisms after mechanical stimulation. The research on mechanotransduction is fairly complex, not only because of the difficulty in ensuring functional conditions but also because the type of cell response is determined by the intensity, rate and frequency of the mechanical forces applied on the system.

The complex mechanisms behind osteoblast differentiation and the interactions of osteoblasts with osteocytes and osteoclasts, indicate our incomplete knowledge on the signaling pathways that govern bone biology. Therefore, there is an abundance of molecules whose action must be identified and interpreted. The mechanisms through which osteocytes receive and interpret mechanical stimuli of different characteristics and transmit it to osteoblasts remains unknown, as remain the mechanisms through which osteoblasts coordinate the activation of specific signaling pathways after mechanical stimulation. Therefore, further investigation of the molecular basis of mechanotransduction in bone physiology is needed in order to evaluate the best suited therapeutic strategy to be followed for the treatment of serious bone diseases like osteoporosis and at the same time avoid any side effects that occur with conventional treatment like the administration of pharmaceutical substances.

References

[1] Junqueira, L. C., Carneiro, J. and Kelley, R. O. (1998). *Basic Histology* (9 ed). Stamford, Connecticut.

[2] Ducy, P., Schinke, T. and Karsenty, G. (2000). The osteoblast: a sophisticated fibroblast under central surveillance. *Science*, 289, 1501-1504.

[3] Dodds, P. R., Caride, V. J. and Lytton, B. (1981). The role of vertebral veins in the dissemination of prostatic carcinoma. *J. Urol.*, 126, 753-755.

[4] Ikeda, T., Kasai, M., Utsuyama, M., and Hirokawa, K. (2001). Determination of three isoforms of the receptor activator of nuclear factor-kappaB ligand and their differential expression in bone and thymus. *Endocrinology*, 142, 1419-1426.

[5] Paget, S. (1989). The distribution of secondary growths in cancer of the breast. *Cancer Metastasis Rev.*, 8, 98-101.

[6] Papachristou, D. J., Basdra, E. K. and Papavassiliou, A. G. (2012). Bone metastases: molecular mechanisms and novel therapeutic interventions. *Med. Res. Rev.*, 32, 611-636.

[7] Ducy, P. and Karsenty, G. (1998). Genetic control of cell differentiation in the skeleton. *Curr. Opin. Cell Biol.*, 10, 614-619.

[8] Aubin, J. E. (1998). Advances in the osteoblast lineage. *Biochem. Cell Biol.*, 76, 899-910.

[9] Bikle, D. D. (2008). Integrins, insulin like growth factors, and the skeletal response to load. *Osteoporos Int.*, 19, 1237-1246.

[10] Papachroni, K. K., Karatzas, D. N., Papavassiliou, K. A., Basdra, E. K., and Papavassiliou, A. G. (2009). Mechanotransduction in osteoblast regulation and bone disease. *Trends Mol. Med.*, 15, 208-216.

[11] Zelzer, E. and Olsen, B. R. (2005). Multiple roles of vascular endothelial growth factor (VEGF) in skeletal development, growth, and repair. *Curr. Top Dev. Biol.*, 65, 169-187.

[12] Kim, S. J., Kim, S. Y., Kwon, C. H., and Kim, Y. K. (2007). Differential effect of FGF and PDGF on cell proliferation and migration in osteoblastic cells. *Growth Factors*, 25, 77-86.

[13] Ducy, P., Zhang, R., Geoffroy, V., Ridall, A. L., and Karsenty, G. (1997). Osf2/Cbfa1: a transcriptional activator of osteoblast differentiation. *Cell*, 89, 747-754.

[14] Harada, H., Tagashira, S., Fujiwara, M., Ogawa, S., Katsumata, T., Yamaguchi, A., et al. (1999). Cbfa1 isoforms exert functional differences in osteoblast differentiation. *J. Biol. Chem.*, 274, 6972-6978.

[15] Jimenez, M. J., Balbin, M., Lopez, J. M., Alvarez, J., Komori, T., and Lopez-Otin, C. (1999). Collagenase 3 is a target of Cbfa1, a transcription factor of the runt gene family involved in bone formation. *Mol. Cell Biol.*, 19, 4431-4442.

[16] Ziros, P. G., Basdra, E. K. and Papavassiliou, A. G. (2008). Runx2: of bone and stretch. *Int. J. Biochem. Cell Biol.*, 40, 1659-1663.

[17] Ducy, P. and Karsenty, G. (1995). Two distinct osteoblast-specific cis-acting elements control expression of a mouse osteocalcin gene. *Mol. Cell Biol.*, 15, 1858-1869.

[18] Geoffroy, V., Ducy, P. and Karsenty, G. (1995). A PEBP2 alpha/AML-1-related factor increases osteocalcin promoter activity through its binding to an osteoblast-specific cis-acting element. *J. Biol. Chem.*, 270, 30973-30979.

[19] Merriman, H. L., van Wijnen, A. J., Hiebert, S., Bidwell, J. P., Fey, E., Lian, J., et al. (1995). The tissue-specific nuclear matrix protein, NMP-2, is a member of the AML/CBF/PEBP2/runt domain transcription factor family: interactions with the osteocalcin gene promoter. *Biochemistry*, 34, 13125-13132.

[20] Marie, P. J. (2008). Transcription factors controlling osteoblastogenesis. *Arch. Biochem. Biophys.*, 473, 98-105.

[21] Huang, G., Shigesada, K., Ito, K., Wee, H. J., Yokomizo, T., and Ito, Y. (2001). Dimerization with PEBP2beta protects RUNX1/AML1 from ubiquitin-proteasome-mediated degradation. *EMBO J.*, *20*, 723-733.

[22] Zhang, Y. W., Bae, S. C., Takahashi, E., and Ito, Y. (1997). The cDNA cloning of the transcripts of human PEBP2alphaA/CBFA1 mapped to 6p12.3-p21.1, the locus for cleidocranial dysplasia. *Oncogene*, 15, 367-371.

[23] Li, Y. L. and Xiao, Z. S. (2007). Advances in Runx2 regulation and its isoforms. *Med. Hypotheses*, 68, 169-175.

[24] Xiao, Z. S., Hjelmeland, A. B. and Quarles, L. D. (2004). Selective deficiency of the "bone-related" Runx2-II unexpectedly preserves osteoblast-mediated skeletogenesis. *J. Biol. Chem.*, 279, 20307-20313.

[25] Ducy, P., Starbuck, M., Priemel, M., Shen, J., Pinero, G., Geoffroy, V., et al. (1999). A Cbfa1-dependent genetic pathway controls bone formation beyond embryonic development. *Genes Dev.*, 13, 1025-1036.

[26] Otto, F., Thornell, A. P., Crompton, T., Denzel, A., Gilmour, K. C., Rosewell, I. R., et al. (1997). Cbfa1, a candidate gene for cleidocranial dysplasia syndrome, is essential for osteoblast differentiation and bone development. *Cell*, 89, 765-771.

[27] Komori, T., Yagi, H., Nomura, S., Yamaguchi, A., Sasaki, K., Deguchi, K., et al. (1997). Targeted disruption of Cbfa1 results in a complete lack of bone formation owing to maturational arrest of osteoblasts. *Cell*, 89, 755-764.

[28] Geoffroy, V., Kneissel, M., Fournier, B., Boyde, A., and Matthias, P. (2002). High bone resorption in adult aging transgenic mice overexpressing cbfa1/runx2 in cells of the osteoblastic lineage. *Mol. Cell Biol.*, 22, 6222-6233.

[29] Liu, W., Toyosawa, S., Furuichi, T., Kanatani, N., Yoshida, C., Liu, Y., et al. (2001). Overexpression of Cbfa1 in osteoblasts inhibits osteoblast maturation and causes osteopenia with multiple fractures. *J. Cell Biol.*, 155, 157-166.

[30] Ziros, P. G., Georgakopoulos, T., Habeos, I., Basdra, E. K., and Papavassiliou, A. G. (2004). Growth hormone attenuates the transcriptional activity of Runx2 by facilitating its physical association with Stat3beta. *J. Bone Miner. Res.*, 19, 1892-1904.

[31] Alliston, T., Choy, L., Ducy, P., Karsenty, G., and Derynck, R. (2001). TGF-beta-induced repression of CBFA1 by Smad3 decreases cbfa1 and osteocalcin expression and inhibits osteoblast differentiation. *EMBO J.*, 20, 2254-2272.

[32] D'Alonzo, R. C., Selvamurugan, N., Karsenty, G., and Partridge, N. C. (2002). Physical interaction of the activator protein-1 factors c-Fos and c-Jun with Cbfa1 for collagenase-3 promoter activation. *J. Biol. Chem.*, 277, 816-822.

[33] Hanai, J., Chen, L. F., Kanno, T., Ohtani-Fujita, N., Kim, W. Y., Guo, W. H., et al. (1999). Interaction and functional cooperation of PEBP2/CBF with Smads. Synergistic induction of the immunoglobulin germline Calpha promoter. *J. Biol. Chem.*, 274, 31577-31582.

[34] Nakashima, K., Zhou, X., Kunkel, G., Zhang, Z., Deng, J. M., Behringer, R. R., et al. (2002). The novel zinc finger-containing transcription factor osterix is required for osteoblast differentiation and bone formation. *Cell*, 108, 17-29.

[35] Koga, T., Matsui, Y., Asagiri, M., Kodama, T., de Crombrugghe, B., Nakashima, K., et al. (2005). NFAT and Osterix cooperatively regulate bone formation. *Nat. Med.*, 11, 880-885.

[36] Wang, X., Kua, H. Y., Hu, Y., Guo, K., Zeng, Q., Wu, Q., et al. (2006). p53 functions as a negative regulator of osteoblastogenesis, osteoblast-dependent osteoclastogenesis, and bone remodeling. *J. Cell Biol.*, 172, 115-125.

[37] Glass, D. A., 2nd and Karsenty, G. (2007). In vivo analysis of Wnt signaling in bone. *Endocrinology*, 148, 2630-2634.

[38] Xiao, G., Jiang, D., Ge, C., Zhao, Z., Lai, Y., Boules, H., et al. (2005). Cooperative interactions between activating transcription factor 4 and Runx2/Cbfa1 stimulate osteoblast-specific osteocalcin gene expression. *J. Biol. Chem.*, 280, 30689-30696.

[39] Yang, X., Matsuda, K., Bialek, P., Jacquot, S., Masuoka, H. C., Schinke, T., et al. (2004). ATF4 is a substrate of RSK2 and an essential regulator of osteoblast biology; implication for Coffin-Lowry Syndrome. *Cell*, 117, 387-398.

[40] Levi, G., Mantero, S., Barbieri, O., Cantatore, D., Paleari, L., Beverdam, A., et al. (2006). Msx1 and Dlx5 act independently in development of craniofacial skeleton, but converge on the regulation of Bmp signaling in palate formation. *Mech. Dev.*, 123, 3-16.

[41] Holleville, N., Mateos, S., Bontoux, M., Bollerot, K., and Monsoro-Burq, A. H. (2007). Dlx5 drives Runx2 expression and osteogenic differentiation in developing cranial suture mesenchyme. *Dev. Biol.*, 304, 860-874.
[42] Samee, N., Geoffroy, V., Marty, C., Schiltz, C., Vieux-Rochas, M., Levi, G., et al. (2008). Dlx5, a positive regulator of osteoblastogenesis, is essential for osteoblast-osteoclast coupling. *Am. J. Pathol.*, 173, 773-780.
[43] Pratap, J., Galindo, M., Zaidi, S. K., Vradii, D., Bhat, B. M., Robinson, J. A., et al. (2003). Cell growth regulatory role of Runx2 during proliferative expansion of preosteoblasts. *Cancer Res.*, 63, 5357-5362.
[44] Stein, G. S., Lian, J. B., van Wijnen, A. J., Stein, J. L., Montecino, M., Javed, A., et al. (2004). Runx2 control of organization, assembly and activity of the regulatory machinery for skeletal gene expression. *Oncogene*, 23, 4315-4329.
[45] Raisz, L. G. (1999). Physiology and pathophysiology of bone remodeling. *Clin. Chem.*, 45, 1353-1358.
[46] Raggatt, L. J. and Partridge, N. C. (2010). Cellular and molecular mechanisms of bone remodeling. *J. Biol. Chem.*, 285, 25103-25108.
[47] Arai, H., Miyamoto, K., Taketani, Y., Yamamoto, H., Iemori, Y., Morita, K., et al. (1997). A vitamin D receptor gene polymorphism in the translation initiation codon: effect on protein activity and relation to bone mineral density in Japanese women. *J. Bone Miner. Res.*, 12, 915-921.
[48] Liu, B. Y., Guo, J., Lanske, B., Divieti, P., Kronenberg, H. M. and Bringhurst, F. R. (1998). Conditionally immortalized murine bone marrow stromal cells mediate parathyroid hormone-dependent osteoclastogenesis in vitro. *Endocrinology*, 139, 1952-1964.
[49] Ohlsson, C., Bengtsson, B. A., Isaksson, O. G., Andreassen, T. T. and Slootweg, M. C. (1998). Growth hormone and bone. *Endocr. Rev.*, 19, 55-79.
[50] Clowes, J. A., Riggs, B. L. and Khosla, S. (2005). The role of the immune system in the pathophysiology of osteoporosis. *Immunol. Rev.*, 208, 207-227.
[51] McCormick, R. K. (2007). Osteoporosis: integrating biomarkers and other diagnostic correlates into the management of bone fragility. *Altern. Med. Rev.*, 12, 113-145.
[52] Boyce, B. F. and Xing, L. (2008). Functions of RANKL/RANK/OPG in bone modeling and remodeling. *Arch. Biochem. Biophys.*, 473, 139-146.
[53] Bucaro, M. A., Fertala, J., Adams, C. S., Steinbeck, M., Ayyaswamy, P., Mukundakrishnan, K., et al. (2004). Bone cell survival in microgravity: evidence that modeled microgravity increases osteoblast sensitivity to apoptogens. *Ann. N Y Acad. Sci.*, 1027, 64-73.
[54] Krane, S. M. (2005). Identifying genes that regulate bone remodeling as potential therapeutic targets. *J. Exp. Med.*, 201, 841-843.
[55] Ehrlich, P. J. and Lanyon, L. E. (2002). Mechanical strain and bone cell function: a review. *Osteoporos. Int.*, 13, 688-700.
[56] Forwood, M. R., Owan, I., Takano, Y., and Turner, C. H. (1996). Increased bone formation in rat tibiae after a single short period of dynamic loading in vivo. *Am. J. Physiol.*, 270, E419-423.
[57] Hatton, J. P., Pooran, M., Li, C. F., Luzzio, C., and Hughes-Fulford, M. (2003). A short pulse of mechanical force induces gene expression and growth in MC3T3-E1 osteoblasts via an ERK 1/2 pathway. *J. Bone Miner. Res.*, 18, 58-66.

[58] Turner, C. H. (1998). Three rules for bone adaptation to mechanical stimuli. *Bone*, 23, 399-407.

[59] Robling, A. G., Hinant, F. M., Burr, D. B., and Turner, C. H. (2002). Improved bone structure and strength after long-term mechanical loading is greatest if loading is separated into short bouts. *J. Bone Miner. Res.*, 17, 1545-1554.

[60] Raab-Cullen, D. M., Akhter, M. P., Kimmel, D. B., and Recker, R. R. (1994). Periosteal bone formation stimulated by externally induced bending strains. *J. Bone Miner. Res.*, 9, 1143-1152.

[61] Rubin, C. T., Gross, T. S., McLeod, K. J., and Bain, S. D. (1995). Morphologic stages in lamellar bone formation stimulated by a potent mechanical stimulus. *J. Bone Miner. Res.*, 10, 488-495.

[62] Agarwal, S., Long, P., Seyedain, A., Piesco, N., Shree, A. and Gassner, R. (2003). A central role for the nuclear factor-kappaB pathway in anti-inflammatory and proinflammatory actions of mechanical strain. *FASEB J.*, 17, 899-901.

[63] Yamamoto, T., Kita, M., Kimura, I., Oseko, F., Terauchi, R., Takahashi, K., et al. (2006). Mechanical stress induces expression of cytokines in human periodontal ligament cells. *Oral. Dis.*, 12, 171-175.

[64] Murray, D. W. and Rushton, N. (1990). The effect of strain on bone cell prostaglandin E2 release: a new experimental method. *Calcif. Tissue Int.*, 47, 35-39.

[65] Kim, T., Handa, A., Iida, J., and Yoshida, S. (2007). RANKL expression in rat periodontal ligament subjected to a continuous orthodontic force. *Arch. Oral. Biol.*, 52, 244-250.

[66] Tsuji, K., Uno, K., Zhang, G. X., and Tamura, M. (2004). Periodontal ligament cells under intermittent tensile stress regulate mRNA expression of osteoprotegerin and tissue inhibitor of matrix metalloprotease-1 and -2. *J. Bone Miner. Metab.*, 22, 94-103.

[67] Wada, T., Nakashima, T., Hiroshi, N., and Penninger, J. M. (2006). RANKL-RANK signaling in osteoclastogenesis and bone disease. *Trends Mol. Med.*, 12, 17-25.

[68] Cheng, M., Zaman, G., Rawlinson, S. C., Mohan, S., Baylink, D. J., and Lanyon, L. E. (1999). Mechanical strain stimulates ROS cell proliferation through IGF-II and estrogen through IGF-I. *J. Bone Miner. Res.*, 14, 1742-1750.

[69] Cillo, J. E., Jr., Gassner, R., Koepsel, R. R., and Buckley, M. J. (2000). Growth factor and cytokine gene expression in mechanically strained human osteoblast-like cells: implications for distraction osteogenesis. *Oral Surg. Oral Med. Oral Pathol. Oral Radiol. Endod.*, 90, 147-154.

[70] Gosain, A. K., Song, L. S., Santoro, T., Weihrauch, D., Bosi, B. O., Corrao, M. A., et al. (2000). Effects of transforming growth factor-beta and mechanical strain on osteoblast cell counts: an in vitro model for distraction osteogenesis. *Plast. Reconstr. Surg.*, 105, 130-136.

[71] Lean, J. M., Jagger, C. J., Chambers, T. J., and Chow, J. W. (1995). Increased insulin-like growth factor I mRNA expression in rat osteocytes in response to mechanical stimulation. *Am. J. Physiol.*, 268, E318-327.

[72] Harter, L. V., Hruska, K. A. and Duncan, R. L. (1995). Human osteoblast-like cells respond to mechanical strain with increased bone matrix protein production independent of hormonal regulation. *Endocrinology*, 136, 528-535.

[73] Jones, D. B., Nolte, H., Scholubbers, J. G., Turner, E., and Veltel, D. (1991). Biochemical signal transduction of mechanical strain in osteoblast-like cells. *Biomaterials*, 12, 101-110.

[74] Kletsas, D., Basdra, E. K. and Papavassiliou, A. G. (1998). Mechanical stress induces DNA synthesis in PDL fibroblasts by a mechanism unrelated to autocrine growth factor action. *FEBS Lett.*, 430, 358-362.

[75] Duncan, R. L. and Hruska, K. A. (1994). Chronic, intermittent loading alters mechanosensitive channel characteristics in osteoblast-like cells. *Am. J. Physiol.*, 267, F909-916.

[76] Carvalho, R. S., Scott, J. E. and Yen, E. H. (1995). The effects of mechanical stimulation on the distribution of beta 1 integrin and expression of beta 1-integrin mRNA in TE-85 human osteosarcoma cells. *Arch. Oral Biol.*, 40, 257-264.

[77] Ziambaras, K., Lecanda, F., Steinberg, T. H., and Civitelli, R. (1998). Cyclic stretch enhances gap junctional communication between osteoblastic cells. *J. Bone Miner. Res.*, 13, 218-228.

[78] Shyy, J. Y. and Chien, S. (1997). Role of integrins in cellular responses to mechanical stress and adhesion. *Curr. Opin. Cell Biol.*, 9, 707-713.

[79] Knudsen, H. L. and Frangos, J. A. (1997). Role of cytoskeleton in shear stress-induced endothelial nitric oxide production. *Am. J. Physiol.*, 273, H347-355.

[80] Howe, A., Aplin, A. E., Alahari, S. K., and Juliano, R. L. (1998). Integrin signaling and cell growth control. *Curr. Opin. Cell Biol.*, 10, 220-231.

[81] Van Aelst, L. and D'Souza-Schorey, C. (1997). Rho GTPases and signaling networks. *Genes Dev.*, 11, 2295-2322.

[82] Basdra, E. K., Papavassiliou, A. G. and Huber, L. A. (1995). Rab and rho GTPases are involved in specific response of periodontal ligament fibroblasts to mechanical stretching. *Biochim. Biophys. Acta*, 1268, 209-213.

[83] Davis, R. J. (1994). MAPKs: new JNK expands the group. *Trends Biochem. Sci.*, 19, 470-473.

[84] Gupta, S., Barrett, T., Whitmarsh, A. J., Cavanagh, J., Sluss, H. K., Derijard, B., et al. (1996). Selective interaction of JNK protein kinase isoforms with transcription factors. *EMBO J.*, 15, 2760-2770.

[85] Ip, Y. T. and Davis, R. J. (1998). Signal transduction by the c-Jun N-terminal kinase (JNK)--from inflammation to development. *Curr. Opin. Cell Biol.*, 10, 205-219.

[86] Schmidt, C., Pommerenke, H., Durr, F., Nebe, B., and Rychly, J. (1998). Mechanical stressing of integrin receptors induces enhanced tyrosine phosphorylation of cytoskeletally anchored proteins. *J. Biol. Chem.*, 273, 5081-5085.

[87] Takeuchi, Y., Suzawa, M., Kikuchi, T., Nishida, E., Fujita, T., and Matsumoto, T. (1997). Differentiation and transforming growth factor-beta receptor down-regulation by collagen-alpha2beta1 integrin interaction is mediated by focal adhesion kinase and its downstream signals in murine osteoblastic cells. *J. Biol. Chem.*, 272, 29309-29316.

[88] Karin, M. and Hunter, T. (1995). Transcriptional control by protein phosphorylation: signal transmission from the cell surface to the nucleus. *Curr. Biol.*, 5, 747-757.

[89] Franceschi, R. T. (1999). The developmental control of osteoblast-specific gene expression: role of specific transcription factors and the extracellular matrix environment. *Crit. Rev. Oral Biol. Med.*, 10, 40-57.

[90] Rodan, G. A. and Noda, M. (1991). Gene expression in osteoblastic cells. *Crit. Rev. Eukaryot Gene Expr.*, 1, 85-98.

[91] Stein, G. S., Lian, J. B., Stein, J. L., Van Wijnen, A. J., and Montecino, M. (1996). Transcriptional control of osteoblast growth and differentiation. *Physiol. Rev.*, 76, 593-629.

[92] Carter-Su, C., King, A. P., Argetsinger, L. S., Smit, L. S., Vanderkuur, J. and Campbell, G. S. (1996). Signalling pathway of GH. *Endocr. J.*, 43 *Suppl.*, S65-70.

[93] Huang, Z., Cheng, S. L. and Slatopolsky, E. (2001). Sustained activation of the extracellular signal-regulated kinase pathway is required for extracellular calcium stimulation of human osteoblast proliferation. *J. Biol. Chem.*, 276, 21351-21358.

[94] Lai, C. F., Chaudhary, L., Fausto, A., Halstead, L. R., Ory, D. S., Avioli, L. V., et al. (2001). Erk is essential for growth, differentiation, integrin expression, and cell function in human osteoblastic cells. *J. Biol. Chem.*, 276, 14443-14450.

[95] Hipskind, R. A. and Bilbe, G. (1998). MAP kinase signaling cascades and gene expression in osteoblasts. *Front Biosci.*, 3, d804-816.

[96] Kousteni, S., Han, L., Chen, J. R., Almeida, M., Plotkin, L. I., Bellido, T., et al. (2003). Kinase-mediated regulation of common transcription factors accounts for the bone-protective effects of sex steroids. *J. Clin. Invest.*, 111, 1651-1664.

[97] Xiao, G., Gopalakrishnan, R., Jiang, D., Reith, E., Benson, M. D., and Franceschi, R. T. (2002). Bone morphogenetic proteins, extracellular matrix, and mitogen-activated protein kinase signaling pathways are required for osteoblast-specific gene expression and differentiation in MC3T3-E1 cells. *J. Bone Miner. Res.*, 17, 101-110.

[98] Karin, M. (1995). The regulation of AP-1 activity by mitogen-activated protein kinases. *J. Biol. Chem.*, 270, 16483-16486.

[99] Marshall, C. J. (1995). Specificity of receptor tyrosine kinase signaling: transient versus sustained extracellular signal-regulated kinase activation. *Cell*, 80, 179-185.

[100] Angel, P. and Karin, M. (1991). The role of Jun, Fos and the AP-1 complex in cell-proliferation and transformation. *Biochim. Biophys. Acta*, 1072, 129-157.

[101] Kletsas, D., Basdra, E. K. and Papavassiliou, A. G. (2002). Effect of protein kinase inhibitors on the stretch-elicited c-Fos and c-Jun up-regulation in human PDL osteoblast-like cells. *J. Cell Physiol.*, 190, 313-321.

[102] Kawata, A. and Mikuni-Takagaki, Y. (1998). Mechanotransduction in stretched osteocytes--temporal expression of immediate early and other genes. *Biochem. Biophys. Res. Commun.*, 246, 404-408.

[103] Pavalko, F. M., Chen, N. X., Turner, C. H., Burr, D. B., Atkinson, S., Hsieh, Y. F., et al. (1998). Fluid shear-induced mechanical signaling in MC3T3-E1 osteoblasts requires cytoskeleton-integrin interactions. *Am. J. Physiol.*, 275, C1591-1601.

[104] Raab-Cullen, D. M., Thiede, M. A., Petersen, D. N., Kimmel, D. B., and Recker, R. R. (1994). Mechanical loading stimulates rapid changes in periosteal gene expression. *Calcif. Tissue Int.*, 55, 473-478.

[105] Inaoka, T., Lean, J. M., Bessho, T., Chow, J. W., Mackay, A., Kokubo, T., et al. (1995). Sequential analysis of gene expression after an osteogenic stimulus: c-fos expression is induced in osteocytes. *Biochem. Biophys. Res. Commun.*, 217, 264-270.

[106] Peverali, F. A., Basdra, E. K. and Papavassiliou, A. G. (2001). Stretch-mediated activation of selective MAPK subtypes and potentiation of AP-1 binding in human osteoblastic cells. *Mol. Med.*, 7, 68-78.

[107] Henthorn, M. J. and Leboy P. (1999). *Acid and alkaline phosphatases.* San Diego, CA, ST: Academic Press.

[108] Howard, P. S., Kucich, U., Taliwal, R., and Korostoff, J. M. (1998). Mechanical forces alter extracellular matrix synthesis by human periodontal ligament fibroblasts. *J. Periodontal. Res.*, 33, 500-508.

[109] Searby, N. D., Steele, C. R. and Globus, R. K. (2005). Influence of increased mechanical loading by hypergravity on the microtubule cytoskeleton and prostaglandin E2 release in primary osteoblasts. *Am. J. Physiol. Cell Physiol.*, 289, C148-158.

[110] Celil, A. B. and Campbell, P. G. (2005). BMP-2 and insulin-like growth factor-I mediate Osterix (Osx) expression in human mesenchymal stem cells via the MAPK and protein kinase D signaling pathways. *J. Biol. Chem.*, 280, 31353-31359.

[111] Zhao, G., Monier-Faugere, M. C., Langub, M. C., Geng, Z., Nakayama, T., Pike, J. W., et al. (2000). Targeted overexpression of insulin-like growth factor I to osteoblasts of transgenic mice: increased trabecular bone volume without increased osteoblast proliferation. *Endocrinology*, 141, 2674-2682.

[112] Yoshida, K., Oida, H., Kobayashi, T., Maruyama, T., Tanaka, M., Katayama, T., et al. (2002). Stimulation of bone formation and prevention of bone loss by prostaglandin E EP4 receptor activation. *Proc. Natl. Acad. Sci. US*, 99, 4580-4585.

[113] Ahdjoudj, S., Lasmoles, F., Holy, X., Zerath, E., and Marie, P. J. (2002). Transforming growth factor beta2 inhibits adipocyte differentiation induced by skeletal unloading in rat bone marrow stroma. *J. Bone Miner. Res.*, 17, 668-677.

[114] Ito, Y. and Miyazono, K. (2003). RUNX transcription factors as key targets of TGF-beta superfamily signaling. *Curr. Opin. Genet. Dev.*, 13, 43-47.

[115] Gu, M., Lynch, J. and Brecher, P. (2000). Nitric oxide increases p21(Waf1/Cip1) expression by a cGMP-dependent pathway that includes activation of extracellular signal-regulated kinase and p70(S6k). *J. Biol. Chem.*, 275, 11389-11396.

[116] Kapur, S., Baylink, D. J. and Lau, K. H. (2003). Fluid flow shear stress stimulates human osteoblast proliferation and differentiation through multiple interacting and competing signal transduction pathways. *Bone*, 32, 241-251.

[117] Reijnders, C. M., Bravenboer, N., Tromp, A. M., Blankenstein, M. A. and Lips, P. (2007). Effect of mechanical loading on insulin-like growth factor-I gene expression in rat tibia. *J. Endocrinol.*, 192, 131-140.

[118] Hughes-Fulford, M. (2004). Signal transduction and mechanical stress. *Sci. STKE*, 2004, RE12.

[119] Lee, M. H., Kwon, T. G., Park, H. S., Wozney, J. M., and Ryoo, H. M. (2003). BMP-2-induced Osterix expression is mediated by Dlx5 but is independent of Runx2. *Biochem. Biophys. Res. Commun.*, 309, 689-694.

[120] Skerry, T. M. (2008). The response of bone to mechanical loading and disuse: fundamental principles and influences on osteoblast/osteocyte homeostasis. *Arch. Biochem. Biophys.*, 473, 117-123.

[121] Duncan, R. L. (1995). Transduction of mechanical strain in bone. *ASGSB Bull.*, 8, 49-62.

[122] Mitsui, N., Suzuki, N., Maeno, M., Yanagisawa, M., Koyama, Y., Otsuka, K., et al. (2006). Optimal compressive force induces bone formation via increasing bone morphogenetic proteins production and decreasing their antagonists production by Saos-2 cells. *Life Sci.*, 78, 2697-2706.

[123] Koyama, Y., Mitsui, N., Suzuki, N., Yanagisawa, M., Sanuki, R., Isokawa, K., et al. (2008). Effect of compressive force on the expression of inflammatory cytokines and their receptors in osteoblastic Saos-2 cells. *Arch. Oral Biol.*, 53, 488-496.

[124] Herman, S., Kronke, G. and Schett, G. (2008). Molecular mechanisms of inflammatory bone damage: emerging targets for therapy. *Trends Mol. Med.*, 14, 245-253.

[125] Tang, L., Lin, Z. and Li, Y. M. (2006). Effects of different magnitudes of mechanical strain on Osteoblasts in vitro. *Biochem. Biophys. Res. Commun.*, 344, 122-128.

[126] Cheng, M. Z., Rawlinson, S. C., Pitsillides, A. A., Zaman, G., Mohan, S., Baylink, D. J., et al. (2002). Human osteoblasts' proliferative responses to strain and 17beta-estradiol are mediated by the estrogen receptor and the receptor for insulin-like growth factor I. *J. Bone Miner. Res.*, 17, 593-602.

[127] Lacouture, M. E., Schaffer, J. L. and Klickstein, L. B. (2002). A comparison of type I collagen, fibronectin, and vitronectin in supporting adhesion of mechanically strained osteoblasts. *J. Bone Miner. Res.*, 17, 481-492.

[128] Zhan, M., Zhao, H. and Han, Z. C. (2004). Signalling mechanisms of anoikis. *Histol. Histopathol.*, 19, 973-983.

[129] Xiao, Z. S. and Quarles, L. D. (2010). Role of the polycystin-primary cilia complex in bone development and mechanosensing. *Ann. N Y Acad. Sci.*, 1192, 410-421.

[130] Ziros, P. G., Gil, A. P., Georgakopoulos, T., Habeos, I., Kletsas, D., Basdra, E. K., et al. (2002). The bone-specific transcriptional regulator Cbfa1 is a target of mechanical signals in osteoblastic cells. *J. Biol. Chem.*, 277, 23934-23941.

[131] Lou, J., Tu, Y., Li, S. and Manske, P. R. (2000). Involvement of ERK in BMP-2 induced osteoblastic differentiation of mesenchymal progenitor cell line C3H10T1/2. *Biochem. Biophys. Res. Commun.*, 268, 757-762.

[132] Ducy, P. (2000). Cbfa1: a molecular switch in osteoblast biology. *Dev. Dyn.*, 219, 461-471.

[133] Hess, J., Porte, D., Munz, C., and Angel, P. (2001). AP-1 and Cbfa/runt physically interact and regulate parathyroid hormone-dependent MMP13 expression in osteoblasts through a new osteoblast-specific element 2/AP-1 composite element. *J. Biol. Chem.*, 276, 20029-20038.

[134] Yasuda, H., Shima, N., Nakagawa, N., Yamaguchi, K., Kinosaki, M., Mochizuki, S., et al. (1998). Osteoclast differentiation factor is a ligand for osteoprotegerin/osteo clastogenesis-inhibitory factor and is identical to TRANCE/RANKL. *Proc. Natl. Acad. Sci. US*, 95, 3597-3602.

[135] Granet, C., Boutahar, N., Vico, L., Alexandre, C., and Lafage-Proust, M. H. (2001). MAPK and SRC-kinases control EGR-1 and NF-kappa B inductions by changes in mechanical environment in osteoblasts. *Biochem. Biophys. Res. Commun.*, 284, 622-631.

[136] Liu, J., Zou, L., Zheng, Y., Zhao, Z., Li, Y., Yang, P., et al. (2007). NF-kappaB responds to mechanical strains in osteoblast-like cells, and lighter strains create an NF-kappaB response more readily. *Cell Biol. Int.*, 31, 1220-1224.

[137] Dalagiorgou, G., Piperi, C., Georgopoulou, U., Adamopoulos, C., Basdra, E. K., and Papavassiliou, A. G. (2012). Mechanical stimulation of polycystin-1 induces human osteoblastic gene expression via potentiation of the calcineurin/NFAT signaling axis. *Cell Mol. Life Sci.*, 69, in press.

[138] Dalagiorgou, G., Basdra, E. K. and Papavassiliou, A. G. (2010). Polycystin-1: function as a mechanosensor. *Int. J. Biochem. Cell Biol.*, 42, 1610-1613.

[139] Scott, A., Khan, K. M., Duronio, V., and Hart, D. A. (2008). Mechanotransduction in human bone: in vitro cellular physiology that underpins bone changes with exercise. *Sports Med.*, 38, 139-160.

[140] Basdra, E. K. and Komposch, G. (1997). Osteoblast-like properties of human periodontal ligament cells: an in vitro analysis. *Eur. J. Orthod.*, 19, 615-621.

[141] Seo, B. M., Miura, M., Gronthos, S., Bartold, P. M., Batouli, S., Brahim, J., et al. (2004). Investigation of multipotent postnatal stem cells from human periodontal ligament. *Lancet*, 364, 149-155.

[142] Lekic, P. and McCulloch, C. A. (1996). Periodontal ligament cell population: the central role of fibroblasts in creating a unique tissue. *Anat. Rec.*, 245, 327-341.

[143] Otto, F., Kanegane, H. and Mundlos, S. (2002). Mutations in the RUNX2 gene in patients with cleidocranial dysplasia. *Hum. Mutat.*, 19, 209-216.

[144] Winslow, M. M., Pan, M., Starbuck, M., Gallo, E. M., Deng, L., Karsenty, G., et al. (2006). Calcineurin/NFAT signaling in osteoblasts regulates bone mass. *Dev. Cell*, 10, 771-782.

[145] Pratap, J., Lian, J. B., Javed, A., Barnes, G. L., van Wijnen, A. J., Stein, J. L., et al. (2006). Regulatory roles of Runx2 in metastatic tumor and cancer cell interactions with bone. *Cancer Metastasis Rev.*, 25, 589-600.

[146] Rubin, C., Turner, A. S., Bain, S., Mallinckrodt, C., and McLeod, K. (2001). Anabolism. Low mechanical signals strengthen long bones. *Nature*, 412, 603-604.

[147] Kusumi, A., Sakaki, H., Kusumi, T., Oda, M., Narita, K., Nakagawa, H., et al. (2005). Regulation of synthesis of osteoprotegerin and soluble receptor activator of nuclear factor-kappaB ligand in normal human osteoblasts via the p38 mitogen-activated protein kinase pathway by the application of cyclic tensile strain. *J. Bone Miner. Metab.*, 23, 373-381.

[148] Tang, L. L., Xian, C. Y. and Wang, Y. L. (2006). The MGF expression of osteoblasts in response to mechanical overload. *Arch. Oral Biol.*, 51, 1080-1085.

[149] Rubin, J., Murphy, T. C., Fan, X., Goldschmidt, M., and Taylor, W. R. (2002). Activation of extracellular signal-regulated kinase is involved in mechanical strain inhibition of RANKL expression in bone stromal cells. *J. Bone Miner. Res.*, 17, 1452-1460.

[150] Armstrong, V. J., Muzylak, M., Sunters, A., Zaman, G., Saxon, L. K., Price, J. S., et al. (2007). Wnt/beta-catenin signaling is a component of osteoblastic bone cell early responses to load-bearing and requires estrogen receptor alpha. *J. Biol. Chem.*, 282, 20715-20727.

[151] Iwamoto, J., Takeda, T. and Ichimura, S. (2001). Effect of exercise training and detraining on bone mineral density in postmenopausal women with osteoporosis. *J. Orthop. Sci.*, 6, 128-132.

[152] Kemmler, W., Lauber, D., Weineck, J., Hensen, J., Kalender, W. and Engelke, K. (2004). Benefits of 2 years of intense exercise on bone density, physical fitness, and blood lipids in early postmenopausal osteopenic women: results of the Erlangen Fitness Osteoporosis Prevention Study (EFOPS). *Arch. Intern. Med.*, 164, 1084-1091.

[153] Sengupta, D. K. (2004). Dynamic stabilization devices in the treatment of low back pain. *Orthop. Clin. North Am.*, 35, 43-56.

[154] Augat, P., Simon, U., Liedert, A., and Claes, L. (2005). Mechanics and mechanobiology of fracture healing in normal and osteoporotic bone. *Osteoporos Int.*, *16 Suppl. 2*, S36-43.

[155] Wolf, S., Augat, P., Eckert-Hubner, K., Laule, A., Krischak, G. D., and Claes, L. E. (2001). Effects of high-frequency, low-magnitude mechanical stimulus on bone healing. *Clin. Orthop. Relat. Res.*, 192-198.

[156] Claes, L., Eckert-Hubner, K. and Augat, P. (2002). The effect of mechanical stability on local vascularization and tissue differentiation in callus healing. *J. Orthop. Res.*, 20, 1099-1105.

[157] Patel, M. J., Chang, K. H., Sykes, M. C., Talish, R., Rubin, C., and Jo, H. (2009). Low magnitude and high frequency mechanical loading prevents decreased bone formation responses of 2T3 preosteoblasts. *J. Cell Biochem.*, 106, 306-316.

[158] Li, L., Zhu, Z., Huang, C., and Chen, W. (2008). Ultrasound: a potential technique to improve osseointegration of dental implants. *Med. Hypotheses*, 71, 568-571.

[159] Wei, Y., Xiaolin, H. and Tao, S. (2008). Effects of extremely low-frequency-pulsed electromagnetic field on different-derived osteoblast-like cells. *Electromagn. Biol. Med.*, 27, 298-311.

In: Osteoblasts
Editor: Hugo Scheurer

ISBN: 978-1-62417-806-1

Chapter 2

From Stem Cells to Osteoblast: Therapeutic Potential for Bone Tissue Engineering

***Smitha Mathews*[1] *and Satish Totey*[2*]**
[1]Centre for Cellular And Molecular Biology, Hyderabad, India
[2]Kasiak Research Pvt Ltd, Mumbai, India

Abstract

Stem cell therapies and tissue engineering have opened up a new era of regenerative medicine, promising the replacement or regeneration of any non-functional or damaged body parts. One of the most exciting approaches is, cell-based bone tissue engineering (BTE), which combines living osteogenic cells with biomaterial scaffolds ex vivo to allow the development of a three-dimensional tissue construct. Mesenchymal stem cells (MSC) that can give rise to osteoblasts are widely used in bone tissue engineering and regenerative therapies. The extracellular matrix (ECM) surrounding the cells play significant role in regulating differentiation and development. An ideal scaffold used for BTE should mimic the beneficial properties of the native tissue ECM for tissue regeneration. ECM based scaffolds are reported to support and enhance the differentiation of MSC into osteoblasts and its maturation. The biomimetic surface coating, that mimic in vivo microenvironment, further improves osteoconductivity of implants and scaffolds and is a key for developing functional tissue for various orthopaedic and bone tissue engineering applications. In this chapter, we will review currently available paradigms governing differentiation of MSC into osteoblast for bone tissue engineering and understand the role of extracellular matrices, biomimetic scaffolds and various biomaterials that enhance the osteogenesis for bone tissue engineering.

* Address for correspondence: Satish Totey, PhD; CEO; Kasiak Research Pvt Ltd, Ghodbunder Road, Thane (W) 400610, Maharashtra, India, smtotey@gmail.com; Satish.totey@kasiakresearch.com.

Introduction

Every year, an estimated 9 million fracture cases occurred globally [1]. One of the challenges confronted by clinicians is the repair and restoration of large bone defect from trauma and other bone diseases. Currently, autologous bone graft is considered as the gold standard for augmenting bone regeneration. However, limited source and volume of bone graft as well as donor site morbidity and related complications have led the scientists to develop an alternative treatment to the autologous bone graft that can maintain its effectiveness, minimize its disadvantages, and be made affordable for the global population [2]. Although, autograft or allograft have gained increasing acceptance, it has the drawbacks including harvesting procedure. The extra surgery involved in harvesting autologous bone causes morbidity at the donor site and causes post-operational pain [3-4]. Allograft is worse than autograft, since it has poor degree of cellularity, less revascularization and higher resorption rate resulting in slower rate of new bone formation [5-8]. Conditions such as postmenopausal osteoporosis, cancer and diabetes usually end up with bone defects or bone fractures. These problems require the application of newer technologies like stem cells therapy or bone tissue engineering to correct the defect.

Bone tissue is a dynamic tissue which is highly vascular in nature. Among the many tissues in the body bone has the highest potential for regeneration.Regeneration requires three main ingredients; 1 signalling proteins in the form of growth factors and cytokines, 2 stem cells to differentiate into specific lineage cells and replenish the damaged cells and 3 scaffolding (Figure-1). In vivo bone regeneration involves osteogenic cells originating from bone marrow mesenchymal stem cells, signalling proteins like bone morphogenic protein (BMP), transforming growth factor (TGF-β), platelet derived growth factor (PDGF) and scaffolding material like extracellular matrix biomaterial.

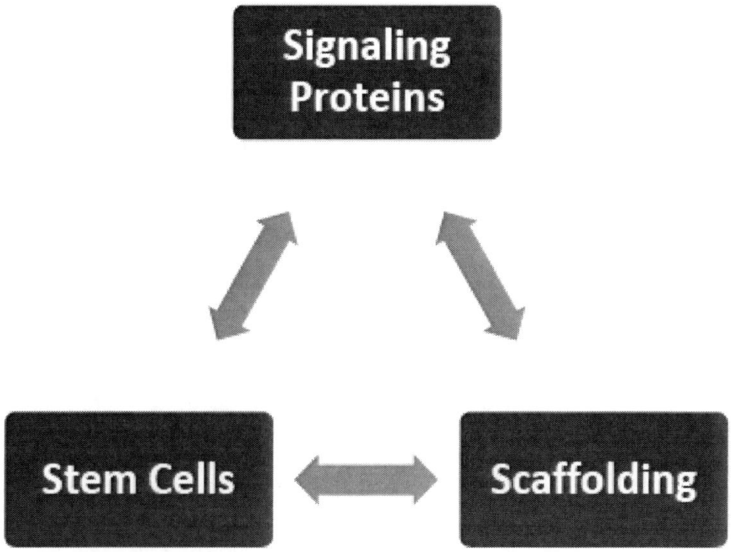

Figure 1. Regeneration trinity. For tissue regeneration requires signalling proteins in the form of cytokines, growth factors and chemo attractant, stem cells and finally scaffolding proteins.

Bone tissue engineering applies these principles of natural bone regeneration to create functional bone tissue constructs in vitro by using osteogenic cells, biomaterial scaffolds, bioactive growth factors, and specialized culture environments [9-10].

The environment supporting in vitro bone formation is created using a combination of biochemical and biophysical signals presented to the cells in a three-dimensional culture system, which allows cell-cell and cell to extracellular matrix (ECM) interactions. The complexity of signalling pathways regulating bone morphogenesis holds significant challenges to engineer a fully viable and functional bone [11].

With the advancement in the field of tissue engineering, significant research was done inidentifying a suitable scaffold material, cell source for reconstructing or repairing the tissue of interest and type of extracellular matrix for cell proliferation and differentiation [12]. The identification of the multi-potential mesenchymal stem cells (MSCs) derived from various adult human tissues has provided exciting prospects for the cell-based tissue engineering and regeneration [13-18]. Since MSCs have the potential to differentiate into osteoblasts, they are widely explored for the development of bioengineered bone constructs using various biomaterial scaffolds. MSCs isolated from human adult bone marrow are considered as the most ideal source of osteogenic cells owing to the ease of isolation; high expansion potential; and the ability to undergo osteoblast differentiation and mineralization [19].

Another best and most exciting approach is a combination of differentiated osteoblast from MSCs and biomimetic scaffolds. Three types of scaffolds can be used for bone tissue engineering, like natural, synthetic and metallic. Scaffold for bone tissue engineering should have properties of biocompatibility; osteoconductivity and osteoinductivity; controlled biodegradability; and high porosity with inter connected pores to enable mass transport, infiltration of cells and interstitial flow of fluids. Apart from promoting osteoblast differentiation, the scaffolds should also promote osteointegration. Generally, scaffolds are considered as the in vitro replacementof the in vivo microenvironment surrounding the cells. So, ideally the scaffold should mimic the in vivo scenario and thus should support cell adhesion, provide cell-cell and cell-ECM interactions and also supply the signals required for cell proliferation and differentiation [20].

Natural scaffold like ECM is an important factor of cellular microenvironment which along with various growth factors plays an important role in cell adhesion, proliferation differentiation and development [21]. ECM is mainly made up of proteins and polysaccharide which has long chains of glycosaminoglycans (GAGs). The biomimetic approach of bone tissue engineering is based on mimicking certain advantageous features of the natural ECM, to facilitate cell recruiting, adhesion, proliferation, differentiation and new bone tissue genesis. So, it is very important to understand the role of various ECM components in MSCs adhesion, proliferation and osteoblast differentiation. Although, many previous studies report the effect of major ECM proteins such as collagen type I, fibronectin, vitronectin and laminin on MSC adhesion, proliferation and osteoblast differentiation, most of these experiments vary in the experimental protocols with non-conclusive and contradictory results. Also, the role of various ECM-GAGs in MSCs adhesion and osteoblast differentiation is a poorly explored area of research.

Since the in vivo environment and conditions which influences the cell behaviour is too complex and less understood; it is not easy to simulate such an environment for an in vitro culture system. In our laboratory, we have carried out various experiments to understand the role of different ECM components and type of scaffold in mesenchymal stem cell behaviour and establish a three dimensional culture system that can closely mimic the in vivo environment for targeted MSC differentiation into osteoblasts.

Mesenchymal Stem Cells

The existences of a different population of stem cells apart from hematopoietic stem cells were first reported by Friedenstein [22]. It was the discovery of mesenchymal stem cells or mesenchymal stromal cells (MSCs) which revolutionized the history of regenerative medicine. MSCs are multi-potent stem cells present in various fetal and adult tissues. They are generally characterized in vitro by their plastic adherence, fibroblast like morphology, expansion and differentiation potential into osteoblasts, adipocytes and chondrocytes.

The mesenchymal and tissue stem cell committee of the International Society for Cell Therapy (ISCT) proposed a set of standards to define human MSC for both laboratory-based scientific investigations and for pre-clinical and clinical studies. They proposed the following three criteria to define MSC: First MSC must be plastic-adherent when maintained in standard culture conditions using tissue culture flasks. Second, more than 95% of the MSC population should express CD105, CD73 and CD90 as measured by flow cytometry. Also, these cells must lack expression (≤ 2% positive) of CD45, CD34, CD14 or CD11b, CD79a or CD19 and HLA class II and third the cells must be able to differentiate to osteoblasts, adipocytes and chondrocytes under standard in vitro differentiating conditions (Figure-2) [23-25]. MSC was initially identified in bone marrow [26], but later have also been isolated from several other tissues such as adipose tissue [27, 28], periosteum [29], tendon [30], synovial fluid [31], skin [32], amniotic fluid [33], umbilical cord [34], umbilical cord blood [35], dental [36], limbal tissue [37], endometrium and menstrual blood [38] brain [39], spleen and heart [40]. MSC has high proliferation capacities, up to 40 population doublings which make them interesting candidate for tissue engineering and cell therapy.

It is hypothesized that, in the adult, these cells are the reservoirs of reparative cells that are mobilized following injury and migrate to the wound site where, in cooperation with local cells, they participate in the repair response. Supporting their stem cell nature is the fact that single cell colonies of MSC express various markers indicating that they are capable of differentiating in vitro and in vivo into cardiac, skeletal muscle, neural cells, tendon and connective tissues. Although, embryonic stem cells (ESC) and MSC are interesting sources as regenerative medicine for clinical application, MSC are preferred because they are ethically non-controversial and present in human body. Both autologous and allogeneic MSC can be used for clinical application since MSC are hypo-immunogenic and have immunomodulatory properties. However it is far from clear that which type of stem cells are most potent and best for therapy. Degree of stemness in adipose tissue and umbilical cord derived MSC was found to be higher than bone marrow and dental pulp derived MSC indicating a higher degree of stemness and self-renewal capacity [41]. It is now known that there are no universal stem cells types or method of delivery that will be universally applicable for stem cell therapy [42].

Gene expression and growth factor profile reflect the source of tissue from where the stem cells have been obtained. This indicates that stem cell heterogeneity is biologically relevant. It has been demonstrated that the gene expression profile and growth pattern of mesenchymal stem cells isolated from various tissue sources are different from each other [43].

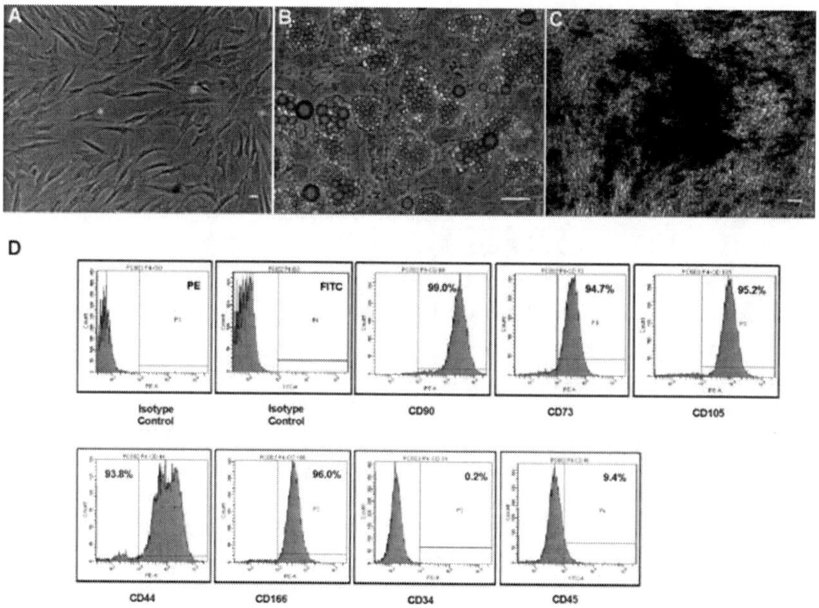

Figure 2. Phase contrast micrograph of mesenchymal stem cells (MSC) showing small slender fibroblast like morphology (A). MSC has ability to differentiate into adipocytes (B) and osteoblasts (C). Immunophenotypically MSCs are positive for CD90, CD73, CD105, CD44 and CD166 but negative for CD34 and CD45 (D). (Scale bar-10μm).

Therefore it is indicated that different tissue sources may generate stem cell products producing different cytokines and growth factors which might be more suited for specific clinical applications.

Bone marrow derived MSC are most extensively studied and widely used stem cells in tissue engineering and regenerative medicine but represents a very small population – 0.001 to 0.01%of the total nucleated cells (24). MSCs are isolated from an aspirate of bone marrow harvested from the superior iliac crest of the pelvis in humans [44, 24]. MSCs are obtained from the mononuclear fraction of the bone marrow by density gradient centrifugation and the primary cultures are usually maintained for 12–16 days. By this time, the non-adherent haematopoietic cell fraction gets depleted and plates will have a confluent adherent population of MSCs.

In order to use MSC in regenerative medicine, it is necessary to isolate and propagate them without the loss of stemness and their differential properties. Many researchers have focussed on developing optimal culture conditions or improving the culture conditions for isolation, propagation and differentiation of MSC for effective clinical applications.

The type of culture media used for isolation and propagation, greatly influenced the viability, growth, characteristics and the differentiation potential of MSC. The major component of the cell culture media are the basal media, fetal bovine serum and L-glutamine. Basal media like Iscove's modified Dulbecco's medium (IMDM), modified eagles medium alpha (MEM-α), Dulbecco's modified Eagles medium low glucose (DMEM-LG), DMEM high glucose (DMEM-HG), DMEM-F12 and knockout DMEM (DMEM-KO) have been used for MSC culture [41, 44, 45, 46].

Studies on evaluation of different basal media led to conclude that DMEM-KO, DMEM-F12 or α-MEM are most suitable and optimal culture conditions for the expansion of MSC as evident from population doubling time, number of population doubling, total cell number, cell surface markers and differentiation potential. MSC cultured in DMEM-KO, DMEM-F12 or α-MEM showed short population doubling time in culture, minimal senescence by β-galactosidase staining and no chromosomal abnormalities [41, 44, 46].

Differentiation of MSC into Osteoblast

Human MSCs are known for their in vitro osteogenic potential [47] and thus hold great promise in bone tissue engineering application [48]. Human MSCs from bone marrow, Wharton's jelly, adipose tissue [49, 50] and dental pulp [51] were also reported to have good osteogenic potential.

When MSC were grown in osteogenic induction media containing ascorbic acid, β-glycerophosphate and dexamethasone, they differentiated into osteogenic lineage and showed mineralization. Osteogenic differentiation can be divided into three phases: (i) the proliferative phase; (ii) the extracellular matrix synthesis and maturation phase; and (iii) the mineralization phase [52].

The proliferative phase is constituted by the lineage committed osteoprogenitor cells which have significant proliferative capacity. This phase is marked by rapid cell proliferation. The osteoprogenitor cells express the cell-growth associated genes H4 histone and cfos [53] and thus undergo frequent mitosis resulting in high cell proliferation. Genes associated with ECM synthesis like collagen type 1α1 (COL1A1), fibronectin and transforming growth factor β (TGF-β) are also expressed in the proliferative phase. Osteopontin (OPN) shows the first peek in expression during this phase.

Extracellular matrix synthesis and maturation phase is marked by the increase in the expression of alkaline phosphatase liver/bone/ kidney (ALPL), integrin binding sialoprotein (IBSP) and COL1A1. ALPL plays an important role in preparing the extracellular matrix for mineralization. This phase is constituted predominantly by pre-osteoblasts. There is minimal cell proliferation in this phase. During this phase, the pre-osteoblasts mature into osteoblasts and there is active synthesis of ECM. Early stage is marked by the presence of COL1, COL3, COL5, fibronectin followed by ALPL.

The final mineralization phase is distinguished by a second peak in OPN expression and the expression of osteocalcin (OCN), IBSP and parathyroid hormone (PTH) receptor by mature osteoblasts. There is no cell proliferation in this phase osteoblasts are the predominant cells.

The alkaline phosphatase (ALP) activity also declines once the mineralization begins. In this phase, the nodule cells begin to mineralize the collagen-based extracellular matrix. 90% of the organic matrix is constituted by collagen type1 and the remaining 10% is non-collagenous proteins (NCP) like OCN, matrix gla-protein (MGP), osteonectin (ON) and fibronectin. Most of these proteins exhibit calcium binding properties. The mineral matrix of bone consists of calcium phosphate in the form of hydroxyapatite (Figure-3).

Detection of intra-cellular calcium and calcium binding proteins and proteoglycans can be detected by Alizarin red S and is ideal for demonstrating the mineralization in the early phases of differentiation whereas, Von Kossa staining mainly demonstrate the calcium in the extracellular matrix and the staining intensity is influenced by the organic matrix.

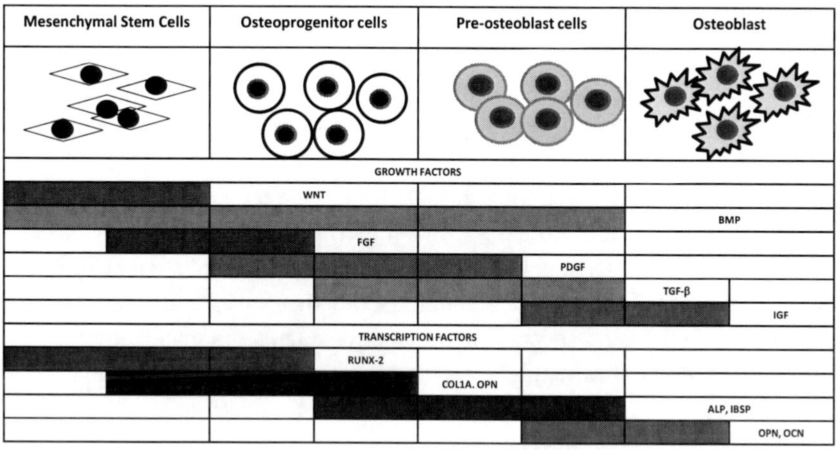

Figure 3. Different phases of osteoblast differentiation and role of growth factors and transcription factors for each stages of differentiation.

Role of Growth Factors and Transcription Factors in Osteoblast Differentiation

Osteoblast differentiation is a strictly controlled developmental process in which numerous extrinsic factors including hormone, growth factors, active osteoblast-specific signalling protein and transcription factors plays crucial role. Plethora of growth factors and proteins controlling cell growth and survivability are constantly up-regulated. Growth factors like, bone morphogenic proteins (BMPs), the transforming growth factor-beta (TGF-b), platelet-derived growth factor (PDGF), fibroblast growth factors (FGFs) and insulin-like growth factors (IGF I and II) are identified to play a significant role in osteogenesis, fracture healing and bone tissue engineering [2,54,55]. Whereas, those proteins functionally associated with osteoblast differentiation and matrix development undergo temporary modulation over time. In particular, the expression of IGF-I, IGF-II, PDGF, FGFR, fibronectin matrix, metalloproteinase, glypican, byglican, osteomodulin, osteonectin, tenascin C, cartilage collagen type VI and XI and bone collagen type I, V, VI and XII increases until immature osteoblast is detectable [20].

BMPs: BMPs are the most extensively studied osteoinductive growth factor. BMP are the proteins grouped into the TGF-β superfamily by virtue of their similarities in protein structure and sequence homology with TGF-β. Their main role is to recruit MSC to the healing site and then differentiate into the osteogenic lineages. They induce the mitogenesis of MSCs and other osteoprogenitors, and there by enhance their differentiation to osteoblasts [56].

BMP especially BMP-2 plays an important role in the expression of alkaline phosphatase and osteocalcin through the mitogen activated protein kinase (MAPK) and nuclear transcription factor like RUNX2/CBAF-1 [57, 58]. BMP has been reported to improve the performance of scaffolds by improving the osteoinduction [59]. Incorporation of BMP-gene in bone tissue engineering applications is another emerging strategy to improve osteoinduction and bone regeneration [60].

FGFs: FGFs are known to promote growth and differentiation of a variety of cells such as fibroblasts, myocytes, osteoblasts, epithelial cells and chondrocytes and known to involve in the bone remodelling process. FGFs appear in the early stages of fracture healing and they act as a mitogen for mesenchymal cells [55]. Transfer of gene encoding basic FGF (bFGF) to MSCs increased their osteogenic potential with enhanced capillary regeneration, thus providing the vasculature necessary for new bone formation [61]. Basic FGF has been used in various BTE applications to enhance osteogenesis [62].

TGF-β: TGF-β is a potent mitogen and chemotactic factor for bone forming cells like MSCs, osteoprogenitors cells, osteoblasts [55]. Autocrine and paracrine stimulation by TGF-β is important in the maintenance and expansion of the mesenchymal stem cells and progenitor of osteoblast. Following TGF-β/BMP induction both the Smad and p38 MAPK pathways converge at the RUNX2 gene to control mesenchymal precursor cell differentiation [63]. TGF-β stimulates cellular proliferation in vitro and is a potent chemotactic stimulator of MSCs and induces the production of bone extracellular proteins such as collagen [64]. Although few BTE studies used TGF-β to improve osteogenesis [65], its osteoinductive potential seems limited, and concern for unforeseen side effects has limited its use in BTE for enhancing bone regeneration [66]. However, it has been reported that TGF-β is a potent inhibitor of terminal osteoblast differentiation and mineralization since it inhibits both cbfa1 transcription factor and osteoblast differentiation [67-69].

VEGF: It is a potent angiogenic factor and expressed in various vascularized tissues. It is commonly found in fracture site and regulate healing process by vascularization through recruitment of endothelial cells. VEGF is a growth factor with angiogenic properties which is widely used for BTE applications to improve angiogenesis and osteogenesis [2]. VEGF is a potent regulator of osteoblast life span in vitro. This autocrine feedback regulates survival of the cells, mediated via a non flt-1 receptor mechanism and expression of Bcl2 anti-apoptotic gene [70].

IGF: IGF family consists of two secreted growth factors like IGF-I and IGF-II where IGF-I is more potent than IGF-II and have effect on bone metabolism and expressed in the osteoblast. They stimulate osteoblast function and bone matrix deposition favouring the synthesis of collagen. However, IGF-I does not influence the differentiation of MSC into osteoblast [71].

PDGF: Platelet derived growth factor is a powerful mitogen for connective tissue cells. Although it can stimulate and synthesized by mesenchymal stem cells and osteoblast like cells, it does not have powerful bone induction properties. It is demonstrated that osteoclast secrete PDGF-BB a chemotactic factor which induces osteoblast chemotaxis via PDGF receptors [72].

Role of Transcription Factor in Differentiation of Osteoblast

The differentiation of mesenchymal stem cells into osteoblast requires a series of cell fate decision controlled by hierarchy of sequential expression of transcription factors. Major transcription factors for osteoblast differentiation are Runx-2, Osterix (OSX), and beta-catenin. Beside these there are other transcription factors including MSX1, MSX2, DLX5, DLX6, ATF4, KNOX20, SP3 and AP1 those are also responsible for osteoblast differentiation [73].

RUNX-2: The first described osteoblast specific transcription factor and the “master switch” for osteoblast differentiation from MSC is Runx-2. This is also known as osteoblast specific factor (OSF 2), polyomavirus enhancer binding factor α (PEBP2αA) or core binding factor α(cbfa1). Runx-2 was shown to be essential for osteoblast differentiation. Mice without Runx-2 gene (-/-) showed no osteoblast and consequently no bone development, but just a cartilage and indicated its importance in the skeletal development. Runx-2 is also expressed in differentiated osteoblast and trans-activate genes involved in the deposition of bone matrix, such as osteocalcin, type-I collagen and osteopontin. This finding further indicates a role of Runx-2 in matured osteoblast [74-76].

OSTERIX (OSX): Osterix (Osx) is one of the few characterized osteoblast genes and thought to regulate numerous osteoblast genes including osteocalcin (OCN), osteonectin (ON), osteopontin (OPN), bone sialoproteins (IBSP) and collagen type-I (COL I) [77, 78]. OSX is essential for osteoblast differentiation and bone matrix deposition and it acts genetically downstream of RUNX2 [79].But interestingly, both OSX and RUNX-2 may act independently of each other.

For example, expression level of OSX remain unaffected in RUNX-2 null mice, similarly level of RUNX-2 is unaltered in OSX null mice [80, 81]. No bone formation occurs in OSX-null mice and their skeleton is composed entirely of cartilage with no osteoblasts and mineral bone matrix [80]. When MSCs were transfected with OSX gene, the over expression of OSX increased MSC proliferation, ALP activity and mineralization *in vitro* [81].

AP-1: AP-1 family of basic lucine zipper transcriptional factor comprises Jun and Fos family proteins and is an important regulatory transcription factor in bone formation and osteoblast function as well as formation and activity of osteoclasts [82]. Several studies have demonstrated an important regulatory role of AP-1 factors, especially Fos related protein in bone formation and osteoblast function as well as formation and function of osteoclast [83]. AP-1 activity in osteoblast is induced by TGF-β/BMP growth factor.

DLX-5 and MSX-2: Osteogenesis is also controlled in part by homeodomain transcription factors that regulate the temporal appearance and location of preosseous tissue [84]. Thus homeodomain proteins may directly mediated osteoblast differentiation by selectively activating or suppressing genes that support osteoblast development.

Dlx5 may not act alone but it may work in conjunction with other transcription factor like Msx-2 [86, 87] Transcription factors like Dlx-5 and Msx-2 are BMP regulated genes and cannot be considered as bone specific genes, but recent studies have indicated role of Dlx-5 and Msx-2 in the differentiation of osteoblast and its maturation [87].

Level of transcription factor Dlx-5 is low at early stage of osteoblast differentiation but this level seems to be increased with the progression of the osteoblast phenotype [88]. However, exact role of Dlx-5 and Msx-2 in regulatory system that determines their function is not currently known.

Scaffolds

Scaffold is a temporary structure that is used as a template for tissue regeneration in tissue engineering. Scaffold consists of matrix and one or several cells types that provide them a tissue specific environment and architecture and guide their growth and tissue regeneration in three dimensions. It also serves as a reservoir of growth factors, cytokines and other nutrients. Scaffold material is biocompatible and possesses the right surface chemistry to promote cell attachment, function and biodegradability. While selecting a biomaterial for tissue engineering applications, apart from the basic qualities like biocompatibility and biodegradability, it is important to understand the role of the particular biomaterial in controlling the behaviour and fate of the cells of interest [89]. Potential materials with these characteristics are either natural scaffolds, synthetic scaffolds or ceramic or metal scaffolds. Biomaterials that mimic native extracellular matrix scaffolding are biomimetic. The biomimetic materials in the musculoskeletal tissues include collagen, proteoglycans, glycosaminoglycan and hyaluronic acid. Other adhesive proteins like fibronectin and laminin also helps in cell attachment to scaffold.

Synthetic biodegradable scaffolds are more commonly used for biomedical engineering field. Most widely used materials for bone tissue engineering that are based on an ester polymer backbone are poly (L-lactic acid) (PLA), [90-93], poly (glycolic acid) (PGA) [94, 95], poly (D-L-lactic acid co-glycolic acid) (PLGA), poly (caprolactone), [96], poly (propylene fumarate) and poly (α- hydroxyl acid) (97, 98). However, US Food and Drug Administration approved PLGA is most widely used scaffold for various clinical application.

Scaffolds like metal and ceramic have been extensively used for bone repair over the last few decades. Metal scaffolds like stainless steel, titanium and cobalt alloy have been extensively used for orthopaedic surgery. Similarly ceramic scaffolds like alumina, zirconia and calcium phosphate are routinely used for bone correction. Hip endoprosthesis is a typical device based on these materials that have remarkably improved the quality of life of many people.

However, both metal and ceramic scaffolds have major disadvantages since they are not biodegradable, difficult to process and difficult to use. But advantage is that they can be used in weight bearing conditions where other natural products are difficult to use.

Therefore, natural and synthetic polymer biodegradable scaffold are now preferred over non-biodegradable metal and ceramic scaffolds [99, 100].

Natural Scaffolds: Extracellular Matrix

ECM is an important part of the cellular microenvironment, which along with various growth factors play a significant role in regulating the differentiation and development [21, 101]. ECM have a major role in deciphering the cell behaviour and function by regulating cell adhesion, differentiation, migration, apoptosis, proliferation, phenotype and growth [102]. Collagen type I, elastin, laminin, fibronectin and vitronectin are the major proteins present in the ECM. Collagen type I is the major protein present in the ECM of bone and it is known to play a significant role in mineralization [65]. It is widely used in bone tissue engineering applications [103, 104]. Collagen coating on various biomaterials has shown to improve cell adhesion [105].

Biomimetic or bio-inspired approach of MSC based bone tissue engineering suggests the potential use of extracellular matrix (ECM) based scaffolds for enhancing differentiation and thereby improving bone regeneration [106-109]. During the osteogenesis of MSC in vivo, the ECM is dynamically remodelled to modulate intracellular signalling during stem cell differentiation [110-112].

In our study, we have seen the effect of four major ECM proteins like collagen type-I, fibronectin, laminin and vitronectin on proliferation and differentiation of MSC into osteoblast lineages. In this study role of the specific ECM proteins at different phases of osteoblast differentiation in terms of osteoblast differentiation associated gene expression and their correlation with alkaline phosphatase expression and mineralization was studied [50]. We observed that early onset of mineralization was observed on collagen type-I coated plates as compared to other ECM or untreated plate (Figure 4). Alizarin and Von Kossa staining for calcium deposition showed that collagen type-I showed higher calcium deposition than other ECM (Figure 4A). We observed a rapid increase in the ALP activity from day 7 to 14 of osteogenic induction and apparent mineralization on all the ECM treated as well as the untreated plates.

The significant role of the ALP gene (ALPL) in initiating and enhancing mineralization was also evident from our osteoblast differentiation associated gene expression studies (Figure 5).

Relative ALPL gene expression at early stage of differentiation was highest on collagen type I, fibronectin and vitronectin treated plates, which showed early onset of mineralization and increased bone matrix secretion. On the contrary, laminin treated plate did not enhance mineralization and bone matrix secretion which was also evidently shown by unaltered ALPL gene expression. This underscores the ALPL associated enhancement of mineralization by the ECM proteins. It appears that collagen type I and alkaline phosphatase are expressed early during the commitment to the osteoblastic phenotype [113]. Our results also showed that increase in ALPL gene expression at early stage of differentiation is critical in mineralization and bone matrix secretion, whereas osteopontin and osteocalcin appears late during osteoblast differentiation and that could be enhanced with the support of appropriate ECM microenvironment. In our study we have shown that collagen type 1, Fibronectin and vitronectin may provide appropriate ECM microenvironment for osteoblast differentiation. However, the significant fold differences observed in the ALPL gene expression was not reflected at protein level. Studies by Gong and Wezeman [114] also supported this discrepancy observed in the ALP expression at the gene and protein level.

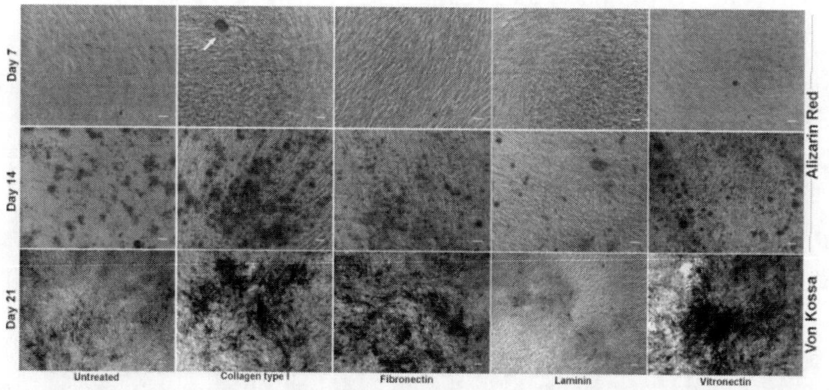

Figure 4. Osteoblast differentiation of MSCs on ECM protein coated plates. The effect of ECM proteins on osteogenesis was assessed by staining (Alizarin Red S and von KossaEarly (day 7) onset of mineralization was observed on collagen type 1 coated plates. Highest calcium deposition was observed on vitronectin treated plates (Scale bar-10μm).

Among the ECM proteins that we have tested in this experiment, collagen type-I was found to be the most appropriate ECM that regulated maximum gene expressions at different stages of maturation of osteogenic differentiation. The gene expression profile on collagen type I treated plate showed significantly high expression of RUNX2, COL1A1, OPN, ALPL, IBSP and OCN at different stages of osteoblast maturation. Recently, several critical transcription factors involved in the process of differentiation in MSC derived lineages have been identified. Osteogenesis of MSC involves RUNX2 which enhance expression of osteogenic genes [115, 81]. Recently, several critical transcription factors involved in the process of differentiation in MSC derived lineages have been identified. Osteogenesis of MSC involves RUNX2 which enhance expression of osteogenic genes [115, 81]. In fact RUNX2 is the first transcription factor required for commitment of the MSCs to osteoblast lineage [116]. High expression of RUNX2 and high ALP activity in the early phase of osteoblast differentiation contributed to the early onset of mineralization with the support of collagen type- I.

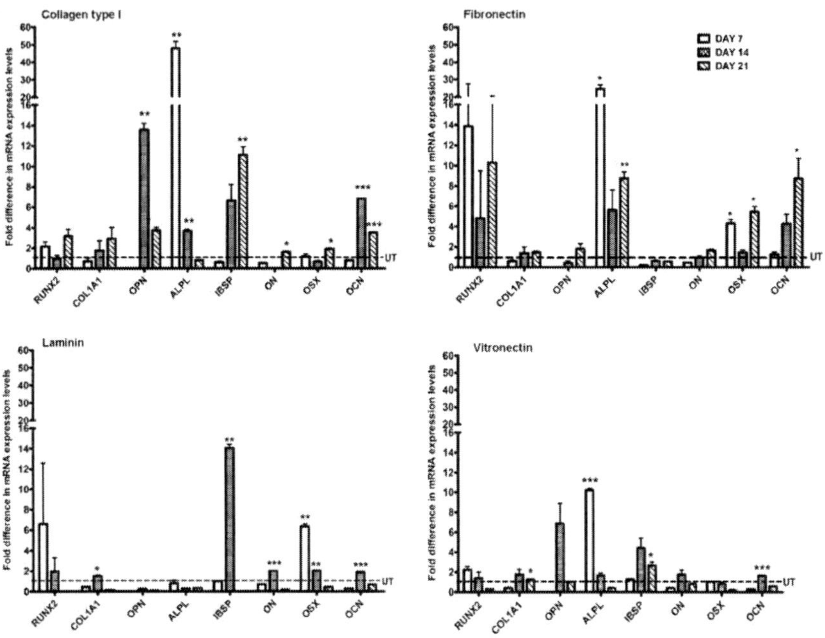

Figure 5. Osteoblast differentiation associated gene expression profile on ECM protein coated plates.UT, untreated.

Kundu and Putnam [117] reported that vitronectin and collagen type I regulated osteoblast differentiation of MSC by two different mechanisms. They suggested that vitronectin stimulated Focal adhesion kinase (FAK) activation which induced osteogenesis possibly by influencing the activity of RhoA. By contrast cells on collagen type I reduced the activation of FAK and increased the activation of ERK and P13K. ERK induced osteogenesis by the activation of RUNX2. There was significantly higher expression level of the collagen type I receptor $\alpha 2\beta 1$ than vitronectin receptor $\alpha v\beta 3$ by MSC. This finding supports the enhanced cell adhesion and proliferation and subsequent early mineralization observed on collagen type I treated plate.

In a similar study, Salasznyk et al. [118] also reported that adhesion of MSCs to collagen type I and vitronectin promoted osteoblast differentiation better than other ECM proteins.

They also found higher mineral to matrix ratio and calcium deposition on vitronectin treated plate than collagen type I treated plates.

The gene expression profile showed that collagen type I, fibronectin, and vitronectin played important role in enhancing differentiation and thereby improving bone regeneration. Among the ECMs that were used in the current experiment, collagen type-I showed maximum up-regulation of osteoblast differentiation associated genes and was proved to be most important protein and known to play significant role in mineralization and osteogenic differentiation.

It is recommended that collagen type I helps in faster and effective bone healing. Vitronectin, which can form ideal bone, could be employed for the surface modification of biomaterials or implants to enhance mineralization. These findings could be helpful in designing biomimetic ECM protein based biomaterial for bone tissue engineering applications.

Glycosaminoglycans (GAGs)

Major part of ECM is also constituted by polysaccharides which have long chains of glycosaminoglycans (GAGs) usually linked to proteins forming proteoglycans. The GAGs interact with various secreted growth factors, chemokines and proteins which regulate cell signalling and differentiation [119].

The major GAGs of fibroblast ECM include: hyaluronic acid (HA), heparin (HEP), heparan sulphate (HS), chondroitin sulphate (CS), dermatan sulphate (DS) and keratan sulphate (KS) [120-122]. The major part of the inorganic bone matrix is made up of the hydroxyapatite and the organic matrix mainly consists of collagens and GAGs; chondroitin-4-sulphate (C4S), DS chondroitin-6-sulphate (C6S) and KS [123]. HA, the only non- sulphated GAG, can bind to cell surface directly through the CD44 receptor and mediate tissue regeneration and repair. The sulphated GAGs, which are rich in negatively charged sulphate groups, can bind to the positively charged amino group of various proteins and growth factors, thus increasing their local availability [124]. Sulphated GAGs are important for bone formation as they bind to most of the growth factors like FGF, BMP, TGF-β, IGF-II, involved in regulating the cells of osteoblast lineage [125]. It has been shown that maintaining aged MSCs in new ECM restored its self-renewal and osteoblast differentiation in mice [126]. Similarly, artificial biomimetic scaffold containing CS has been demonstrated to promote osteoblast differentiation of MSCs more specifically [127]. Osteoblast differentiation is marked by an initial proliferative phase followed by an extracellular matrix synthesis phase and a final phase of mineralization [128, 129]. The osteoblast differentiation experiments with GAGs provided new insight into the role of ECM GAGs in osteogenesis and its regulation. Among the GAGs HA was proved to have the best osteogenic potential followed by heparin, C6S, and DS. The overall histochemical staining for calcium and bone matrix demonstrated the HA surface to be the most preferable condition for osteoblast differentiation and mineralization. There was early onset of mineralization and significantly large amount of mineral deposition with high calcium content on HA treated plates. HA based hydrogels with BMP-2 and MSCs had the highest expression of osteocalcin and mature bone formation with vascular markers [130]. Also there are studies reporting enhanced mineralization, with increased ALP activity and OPN and COL1 expression by human mesenchymal stromal cells on a biomimetic HA based scaffolds [131]. Though there are many studies [132, 133] proving the osteogenic potential of hyaluronic acid, only a few researchers report the possible mechanism of the osteogenesis by HA. A recent study demonstrating the differentiation of MSCs to pre-osteoblasts in the absence of osteogenic supplements in a HA based gel suggested the integrin mediated MSC adhesion and subsequent sequestration of native ECM components and soluble cytokines with osteoconductive properties [134]. This shows the innate osteogenic potential of HA. Another school of thought is that as MSCs possess CD44 on its surface, the CD44-HA interaction is responsible for facilitating the osteogenic differentiation. The CD44 receptor serve as the primary receptor for the ECM hyaluronic acid and regulate both cell-cell and cell-ECM interactions [135]. CD44-HA binding increases the cellular response to BMP7, which activates the Smad-1 signalling pathway inducing osteoblast differentiation through Hoxc-8 [136]. The calcium quantification showed significantly high amount of calcium on DS, C6S, HEP and HA plates with HA showing the highest amount (Figure-6). Whereas von Kossa staining showed very intense staining on HA plate followed by HEP and lower intensities for C6S and DS. This difference between the calcium quantification and staining for calcium clearly indicates the presence of large amount of organic components in the bone matrix of osteoblasts on HA and HEP treated plates. Calcium assay confirmed that all the GAG treated plates except C4S have significant osteogenic potential and formed mineralized bone matrix with good amount of calcium irrespective of the organic components in the extra-cellular deposits, indicating their therapeutic potential in bone fracture healing [19].

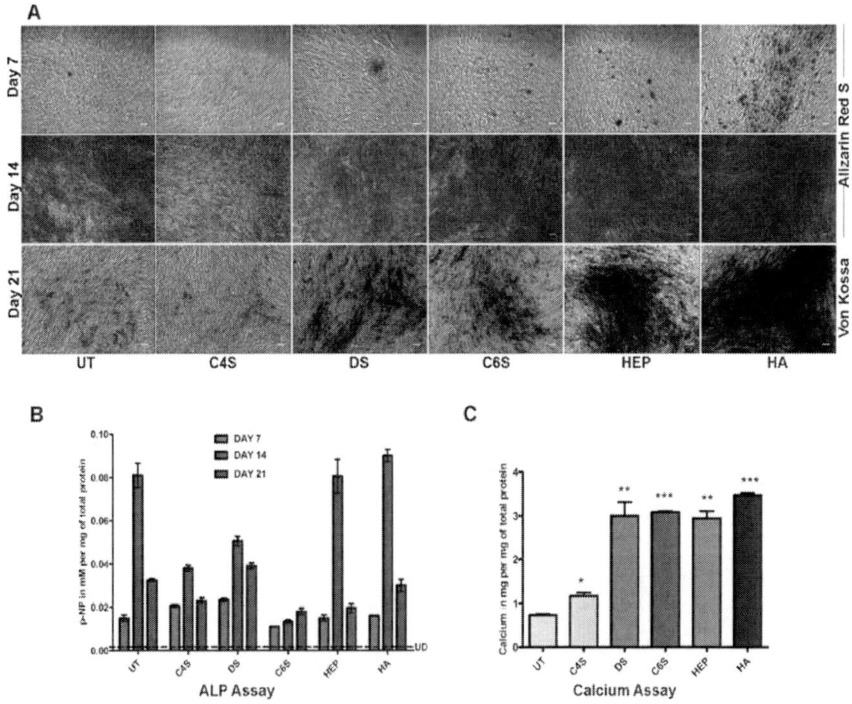

Figure 6. Osteoblast differentiation of MSCs on ECM-GAGs coated plates. The effect of ECM-GAGs on osteogenesis was assessed by staining (Alizarin Red S and von Kossa) for calcium (A) , ALP assay (B) and quantification of calcium (day 21)in the secreted matrix(C). UT, untreated. (Scale bar-10μm).

The osteoblast differentiation associated gene expression profile showed osterix as the key transcription factor responsible for the enhanced bone matrix deposition observed on hyaluronic acid, heparin and chondroitin-6-sulphate coated plates (Figure-7). Genes like osteocalcin, integrin binding sialoprotein, osteonectin and collagen type1 alpha 1 also showed significant up regulation on these plates.

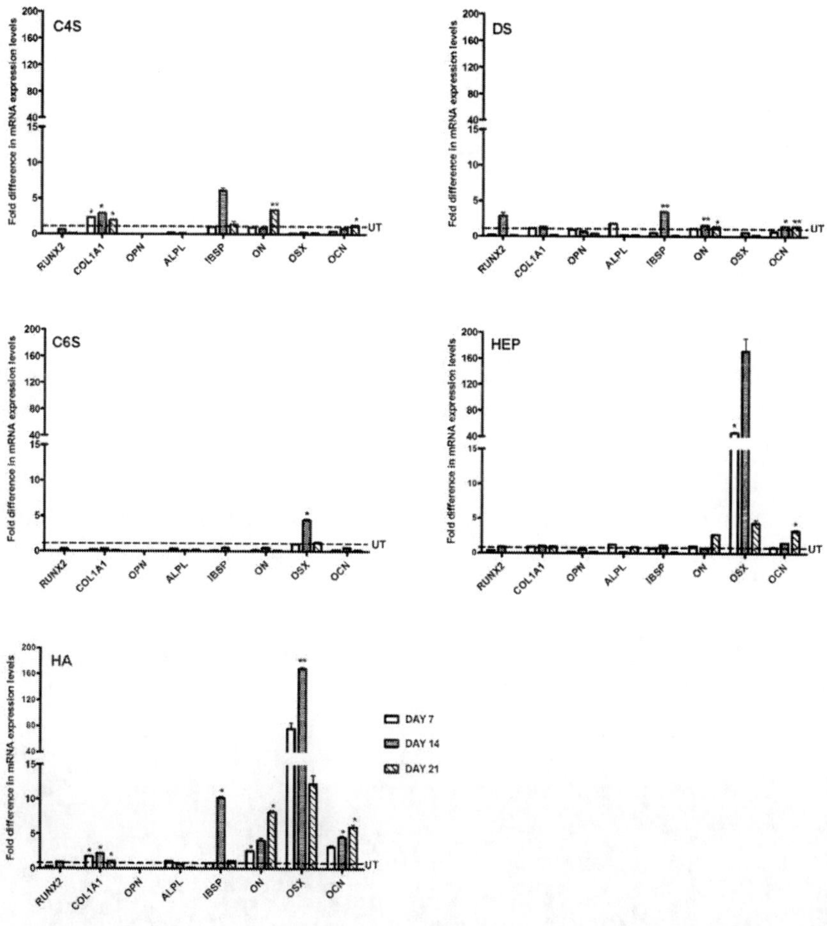

Figure 7. Osteoblast differentiation associated gene expression profile on ECM –GAG coated plates.UT, untreated.

Chitosan Scaffold

An ideal scaffold should mimic the beneficial properties of the native tissue ECM for tissue regeneration. According to Ma [137], the natural ECM or a mirror image of it, need not be the ideal scaffold for tissue engineering applications because tissue engineering should be an accelerated regeneration process compared to the natural development program. So the biomimetic approach of bone tissue engineering can be simply defined as that mimicking certain advantageous features of the natural ECM to facilitate cell recruiting, adhesion, proliferation, differentiation and new bone tissue genesis [137]. The biomimetic approach aims at the induction of bone formation by the implantation of smart, self-inducing biomimetic matrices endowed with shape memory geometries that per se initiate the ripple-like cascade of bone differentiation by induction even without the addition of any exogenous growth factors [138]. Recently, Zhang et al [139] incorporated collagen and the resulted nanofibrous hydroxyapatite/collagen/chitosan composite scaffold significantly increased osteoblast proliferation, alkaline phosphatase expression, and mineral deposition.

Chitosan is a natural biomaterial with a structural similarity to hyaluronic acid of ECM [140, 141]. Though the osteogenic property of chitosan is well established in tissue engineering applications, the exact mechanism is not yet well understood [142, 143].

Excellent properties of chitosan such as osteoconductivity, biocompatibility, biodegradability, low immunogenicity and better mechanical property make it an interesting biopolymer for bone tissue engineering applications [144]. Chitosan scaffolds alone, cannot imitate all the properties of natural bone, while composite scaffolds of chitosan with hydroxyapatite show promise in mimicking the organic portion, as well as the inorganic portion, of natural bone [143]. Chitosan when incorporated with hydroxyapatite showed significant increases in the osteoblastic cell growth [145].

In our study, we examined the optimum coating density of chitosan for MSC culture (146). We have observed that at higher concentration of chitosan (100µg/cm^2) MSC form viable non-adherent cell aggregates, but able to differentiate into osteogenic lineage (Figure-8, 9). Possible explanation for the difference in the cell adhesion properties of chitosan at different coating density may be due to the difference in the adsorbed protein layer on it.

This altered protein layer at higher coating density did not allow the cells to attach to the plate but instead increased the cell-cell interactions resulting in the aggregation of the cells.

It is known that MSC adhere to a biomaterial via the integrin expressed on the cell surface by an indirect mechanism and mediated by the specific serum proteins adsorbed to the material surface [147]. Osteogenic potential of MSC on chitosan treated plated showed significantly higher mineralization and bone nodule formation than the untreated plate.

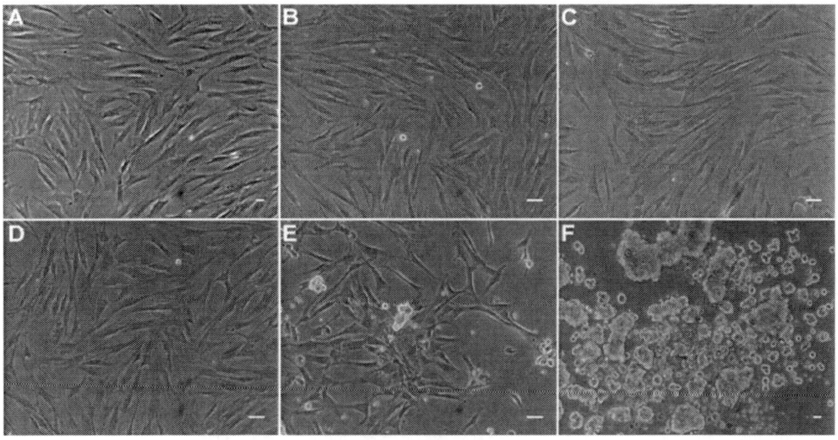

Figure 8. MSCs on chitosan coated plates with different coating densities. Untreated plate (A), 5µg/cm^2 chitosan (B), 10µg/cm^2 chitosan (C), 25µg/cm^2 chitosan (D), 50µg/cm^2 chitosan (E) and 100µg/cm^2 chitosan (F) coated plates. (Scale bar -10µm).

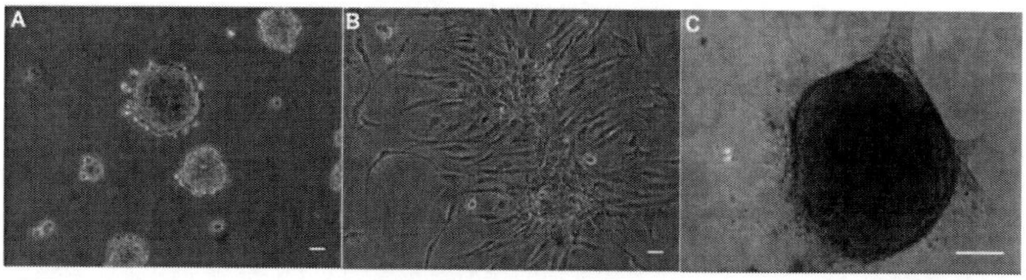

Figure 9. Viable cell aggregates on chitosan (100μg/cm^2) coated plates. Cell aggregates (A) showed viable, adherent population when plated on tissue culture treated plates (B. Alizarin Red S staining confirmed the osteogenic differentiation of the aggregates (C). (Scale bar- 10μm).

Intracellular calcium deposition confirmed by Alizarin Red S staining and extracellular calcium deposition confirmed by von Kossa staining was significantly more in chitosan treated plate. Quantification of calcium in the secreted mineral matrix showed 30% higher calcium on chitosan treated plate than untreated (Figure-10).

Our attempt to understand the osteogenic property of chitosan at a molecular level revealed interesting findings (Figure-11).

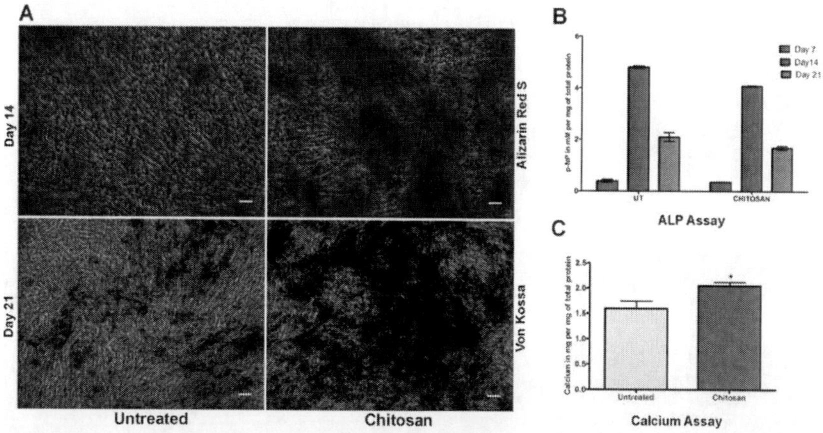

Figure 10. Osteoblast differentiation of MSCs on chitosan coated plates. Alizarin Red S and von Kossa staining for calcium (A), ALP assay (B) and quantification of calcium (day 21)in the secreted matrix(C) were used for evaluating the osteogenic potential. (Scale bar-10μm).

This is the first study showing the relative fold difference in mRNA levels of MSC undergoing osteoblast differentiation on a chitosan coated culture plate. Cells cultured on chitosan coated plate did not show any changes in expression level of RUNX2 gene, the gene responsible for the osteoblast lineage commitment.

But its downstream effecter OSX showed marked increase in expression especially in the initial phases of differentiation and later at the late stage of differentiation. OSX is considered as the key transcription factor required for the differentiation of pre-osteoblasts to mature osteoblasts [148].

Other genes such as COL1A1, ALPL, IBSP, OPN, ON and OCN, which are mostly associated with mineralization showed several fold increase in the level of expression on chitosan coated plates. More COL1A1 expression indicated more calcium binding and thus enhanced mineral matrix deposition on the chitosan coated plates. Both IBSP and OPN genes showed higher expression in the early stages of differentiation on chitosan coated plates. These plates also showed several fold difference in the expression of OCN in the late stage of differentiation as compared to the untreated plate. These findings suggest that chitosan enhances osteoblasts differentiation mainly by up-regulating most of the genes associated with calcium binding proteins which resulted in more bone matrix deposition on chitosan coated plates. The gene expression profile also indicates that chitosan follows the normal pathway of osteoblast differentiation by human mesenchymal stem cells and embryonic stem cells [146, 149, 150].

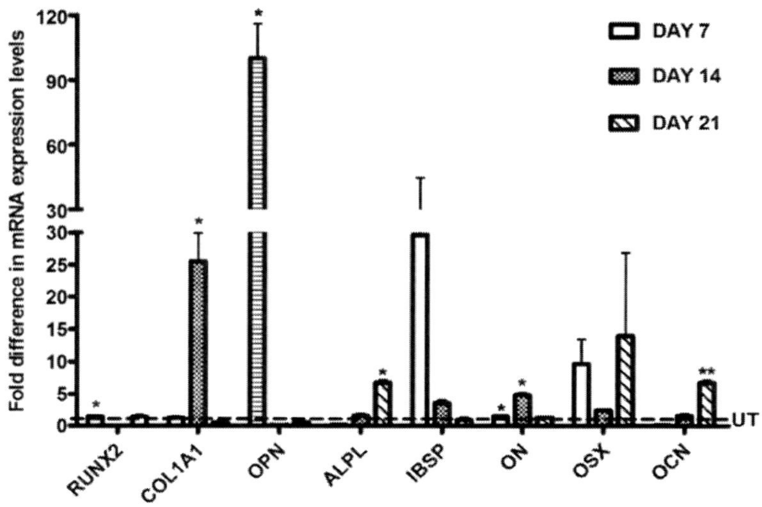

Figure 11. Osteoblast differentiation associated gene expression profile on chitosan coated plates.UT, untreated.

Tripolymer Scaffolds

Based on our previous study we have seen the properties of chitosan scaffold with high osteogenic potential, collagen type-I which enhanced the cell adhesion and bone matrix synthesis and HA that enhanced the mineralization and secreted high calcium containing bone matrix. Composite polymers have always attracted the researchers due to their ability to achieve better mechanical and biological properties than their individual polymers [151, 152]. Based on this data we further studied the synergistic effect of combination of these tripolymers biomimetic coating on osteogenic differentiation and mineralization. Plates were coated with different combination of chitosan: Collagen: HA using mixed polyblend solution or surface modification. To our knowledge, this is a first study using combination of three osteogenic biomaterials for a biomimetic coating of normal tissue culture plates to evaluate their combined effect on the osteogenic differentiation and mineralization of MSC.

Out of several combinations and concentrations the plates which had equal concentration of chitosan: Collagen: HA (1:1:1) showed enhanced mineralization, high calcium deposition, in surface modification method than polyblend method for immobilizing all the three components [153] (Figure-12). Ma *et al* [154] also found the surface modification method more effective than polyblend method for immobilizing hyaluronic acid on the surface of chitosan-gelatin membrane.

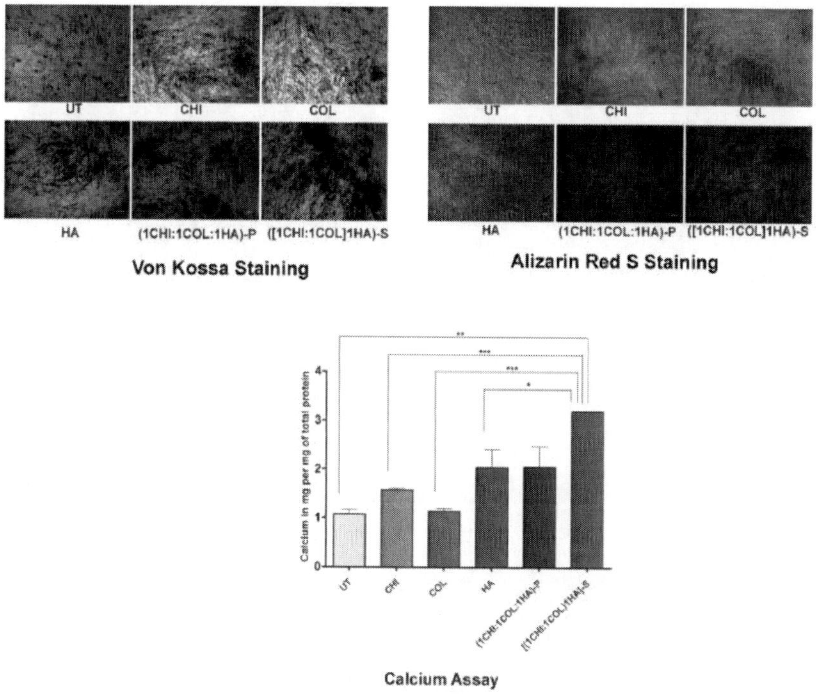

Figure 12. Osteoblast differentiation of MSCs on tripolymer coated plates. UT, untreated; CHI, chitosan; COL, collagen type 1, HA, hyaluronic acid; (1CHI:1COL:1HA)-P, 1:1:1 tripolymer ratio, coating by polyblend method and [(1CHI:1COL)1HA]-S, 1:1:1 tripolymer ratio, coating by surface modification method. (Scale bar-10μm).

Based on this results we developed three dimensional scaffold using chitosan, Collagen and HA for culture system for MSC and osteoblast differentiation. Poor mechanical strength and cell compliance of chitosan has led to the modification of chitosan with other compounds to improve its strength or cell adhesive property or both [155, 156]. The biomimetic modification of chitosan by incorporation of COL (showing excellent MSC adhesion) and HA (having high osteogenic potential) have showed significant enhancement of the osteogenic differentiation of MSC.

Chitosan is a promising candidate that can be used in scaffold design due to its nontoxic properties, affinity to proteins, biocompatibility and biodegradability. While most of the natural polymers are limited in supply, chitosan is abundantly available next to that of cellulose. Despite its favourable biological properties, the weak mechanical strength of scaffold has limited the scope of their application. Various percent compositions from 4 – 12 wt % are utilized to produce a chitosan scaffold that has desirable pore size and porosity properties. Mechanical properties of the scaffold have seen to be increased when chitosan concentration was increased from 1 to 3% (wt/vol) [157, 158]. In bone and cartilage engineering chitosan and HA can be blend together to form 3D scaffold.Oliveria et al. [159] created a bilayer scaffold utilizing the freeze-dry method and pouringa 3% chitosan solution onto a sintered HA scaffold. The scaffolds demonstrated a high connectivity, adequate water uptake and porosity, good mechanical properties and cellular adhesion.

In bone healing process, adequate mineralization of the osteoid is essential for the formation of hard bone and healing of the fracture [160 161]. So our tripolymer combination with adequate osteoconductivity and enhanced mineralization hold great promise for treating bone and cartilage disorders. There are many reports showing enhanced osteointegration by surface modification of titanium implants with collagen type 1 [162, 163]. As our tripolymer coating showed three fold higher MSC differentiation and mineralization than alone collagen type 1 coating, it could be a better option for the surface modification of orthopaedic implants for stem cell based therapy.These findings will be useful in designing chitosan based culture systems for stem cell based bone tissue engineering applications and could be of clinical significance advocating the use of stem cells and chitosan in treating non-union bone fractures and other bone and cartilage disorders.

To conclude, the ECM components indeed modified the adhesion, proliferationand osteoblast differentiation of MSCs in vitro. The difference in the osteoblast differentiation and associated gene expression observed on various ECM componenttreated plates indicates the difference in the regulatory mechanisms. We have successfully developed an ECM based, tripolymer composite consisting of chitosan,collagen type I and hyaluronic acid which holds great promise as a biomimetic coating or scaffold for bone tissue engineering and bone regenerative therapies.

References

[1] Johnell O, Kanis JA. An estimate of the worldwide prevalence and disability associated with osteoporotic fractures. *Osteoporos Int.* 2006; 17(12): 1726-1733

[2] Salgado AJ, Coutinho OP, Reis RL. Bone tissue engineering: state of the art and future trends. *Macromol. Biosci.* 2004; 4(8): 743-765.

[3] Thompson RC Jr, Garg A, Clohisy DR, ChengEY. Fractures in large-segment allografts. *Clin. Orthop.* 2000; 227-35.

[4] Clohisy DR, Mankin HJ. Osteoarticular allografts for reconstruction after resection of a musculoskeletal tumor in the proximal end of the tibia. *J. Bone. Joint Surg. Am.* 1994; 76:549-54.

[5] Damien CJ, Parsons JR. Bone graft and bone graft substitutes: A review of current technology and applications. *J. Appl. Biomaterials* 1991; 2: 187–208.

[6] de Boer HH. The history of bone grafts. *Clin. Orthop.* 1988; 226: 292–298.

[7] Yaszemski MJ, Payne RG, Hayes WC, Langer R, Mikos AG. Evolution of bone transplantation: Molecular, cellular and tissue strategies to engineer human bone. *Biomaterials* 1996; 17: 175–185.

[8] Lane JM, Tomin E, Bostrom MPG. Biosynthetic bone grafting. *Clin. Orthop. Relat. Res.* 1999; 367S: 107–117.

[9] Kneser U, Schaefer DJ, Polykandriotis E, Horch RE. Tissue engineering of bone: the reconstructive surgeon's point of view. *J. Cell Mol. Med.* 2006; 10(1): 7-19.

[10] Bajada S, Mazakova I, Richardson JB, Ashammakhi N. Updates on stem cells and their applications in regenerative medicine. *J. Tissue Eng. Regen. Med.* 2008; 2: 169–183.

[11] Meijer GJ, de Bruijn JD, Koole R, van Blitterswijk CA. Cell-based bone tissue engineering. *PLoS Med.* 2007; 4(2):e9.

[12] Corona BT, Ward CL, Harrison BS, Christ GJ. Regenerative medicine: basic concepts, current status, and future applications. *J. Investig. Med.* 2010; 58(7):849- 858.

[13] Bianco P, Robey PG. Stem cells in tissue engineering. *Nature*. 2001; 414:118-121.

[14] Chatterjea A, Meijer G, van Blitterswijk C, de Boer J. Clinical application of human mesenchymal stromal cells for bone tissue engineering. *Stem Cells Int*. 2010; 2010:215625.

[15] Pal R, Hanwate M, Jan M, Totey S. Phenotypic and functional comparison of optimum culture conditions for up-scaling of bone marrow-derived mesenchymal stem cells. *J. Tissue Eng. Regen. Med.* 2009; 3(3):163-174.

[16] Totey S, Totey S, Pal R, Pal R. Adult stem cells: a clinical update. *J. Stem Cells*. 2009;4 (2):105-21.

[17] Nekanti U, Mohanty L, Venugopal P, Balasubramanian S, Totey S, Ta M. Optimization and scale-up of Wharton's jelly-derived mesenchymal stem cells for clinical applications. *Stem Cell Res*. 2010;5(3):244-54.

[18] Nekanti U, Rao VB, Bahirvani AG, Jan M, Totey S, Ta M. Long-term expansion and pluripotent marker array analysis of Wharton's jelly-derived mesenchymal stem cells. *Stem Cells Dev*. 2010; 19(1):117-30.

[19] Mathews S, Mathew SA, Gupta PK, Bhonde R, Totey S. Glycosaminoglycans enhance osteoblast differentiation of bone marrow derived human mesenchymal stem cells. *J. Tissue Eng. Regen. Med.* 2012 Apr 12. 10.1002/term.1507.

[20] Arvidson K, Abdallah BM, Applegate LA, Baldini N, Cenni E, Gomez-Barrena E, Granchi D, Kassem M, Konttinen YT, Mustafa K, Pioletti DP, Sillat T, Finne-Wistrand A. Bone regeneration and stem cells. *J. Cell Mol. Med.* 2011;15(4):718-46.

[21] Adams JC, Watt FM. Regulation of development and differentiation by the extracellular matrix. *Development.* 1993; 117: 1183-1198.

[22] Friedenstein AJ, Deriglasova UF, Kulagina NN, Panasuk AF, Rudakowa SF, Luriá EA, Ruadkow IA. Precursors for fibroblasts in different populations of hematopoietic cells as detected by the in vitro colony assay method. *Exp. Hematol*. 1974; 2(2):83-92.

[23] Dominici M, Le Blanc K, Mueller I, Slaper-Cortenbach I, Marini F, Krause D, Deans R, Keating A, ProckopDj, Horwitz E. Minimal criteria for defining multipotent mesenchymal stromal cells. The International Society for Cellular Therapy position statement. *Cytotherapy*. 2006; 8(4):315-

[24] Pittenger MF, Mackay AM, Beck SC, Jaiswal RK, Douglas R, Mosca JD, Moorman MA, Simonetti DW, Craig S, Marshak DR. Multilineage potential of adult human mesenchymal stem cells. *Science*. 1999; 284(5411):143-7.

[25] Mafi P, Hindocha S, Mafi R, Griffin M, Kha WS. Adult mesenchymal stem cells and cell surface characterization - a systematic review of the literature. *Open Orthop. J.* 2011; 5(Suppl 2):253-260.

[26] Honczarenko M, Le Y, Swierkowski M, Ghiran I, Glodek AM, Silberstein LE. Human bone marrow stromal cells express a distinct set of biologically functional chemokine receptors. *Stem Cells*. 2006; 24:1030–1041.

[27] Keyser KA, Beagles KE, Kiem HP. Comparison of mesenchymal stem cells from different tissues to suppress T-cell activation. *Cell Transplant*. 2007; 16:555–562.

[28] Zuk PA, Zhu M, Mizuno H, Huang J, Futrell JW, Katz AJ, Benhaim P, Lorenz HP, Hedrick MH. Multi-lineage cells from human adipose tissue: Implications for cell-based therapies. *Tissue Eng*. 2001; 7:211–228.

[29] Nakahara H, Goldberg VM, Caplan AI. Culture expanded human periosteal-derived cells exhibit osteochondral potential in vivo. *J. Orthop. Res*. 1991; 9:465–476.

[30] Salingcarnboriboon R, Yoshitake H, Tsuji K, Obinata M, Amagasa T, Nifuji A, Noda M. Establishment of tendon-derived cell lines exhibiting pluripotent mesenchymal stem cell-like property. *Exp. Cell Res.* 2003; 287:289–300.

[31] De Bari C, Dell'Accio F, Tylzanowski P, Luyten FP. Multi-potent mesenchymal stem cells from adult human synovial membrane. *Arthritis Rheum.* 2001; 44:1928–1942.

[32] Toma JG, Akhavan M, Fernandes KJ, Barnabe-Heider F, Sadikot A, Kaplan DR, Miller FD. Isolation of multi-potent adult stem cells from the dermis of mammalian skin. *Nat. Cell Biol.* 2001; 3:778–784.

[33] Tsai MS, Lee JL, Chang YJ, Hwang SM. Isolation of human multi-potent mesenchymal stem cells from second-trimester amniotic fluid using a novel two-stage culture protocol. *Hum. Reprod.* 2004; 19:1450–1456.

[34] Wang HS, Hung SC, Peng ST, Huang CC, Wei HM, Guo YJ, Fu YS, Lai MC, Chen CC. Mesenchymal stem cells in the Wharton's jelly of the human umbilical cord. *Stem Cells* 2004; 22:1330–1337.

[35] Erices A, Conget P, Minguell JJ. Mesenchymal progenitor cells in human umbilical cord blood. *Br. J. Haematol.* 2000; 109:235–242.

[36] Gronthos S, Mankani M, Brahim J, Robey PG, Shi S. Postnatal human dental pulp stem cells (DPSCs) in vitro and in vivo. *Proc. Natl. Acad. Sci. USA* 2000; 97:13625–13630.

[37] Kim MK, Lee JL, Shin KS, Jung GA, Wee WR, Lee JH, Park KS, Son YS. Isolation of putative corneal epithelial stem cells from cultured limbal tissue. *Korean J. Ophthalmol.* 2006; 20:55–61.

[38] Meng X, Ichim TE, Zhong J, Rogers A, Yin Z, Jackson J, Wang H, Ge W, Bogin V, Chan KW, Thebaud B, Riordan NH. Endometrial regenerative cells: A novel stem cell population. *J. Transl. Med.* 2007; 5:57–66.

[39] Paul G, Özen I, Christophersen NS, Reinbothe T, Bengzon J, Visse E, Jansson K, Dannaeus K, Henriques-Oliveira C, Roybon L, Anisimov SV, Renstrom E, Svensson M, Haegerstrand A, Brundin P. The adult human brain harbors multi-potent perivascular mesenchymal stem cells. PLoS ONE 2012; 7(4):e35577. doi:10.1371/journal.pone.0035577

[40] Hoogduijn MJ, Crop MJ, Peeters AM, Van Osch GJ, Balk AH, IJzermans JN, Weimar W, Baan CC. Human heart, spleen, and perirenal fat-derived mesenchymal stem cells have immunomodulatory capacities. *Stem Cells Dev.* 2007;16(4):597.

[41] Nekanti U, Dastidar S, Venugopal P, Totey S, Ta M. Increased proliferation and analysis of differential gene expression in human Wharton's jelly-derived mesenchymal stromal cells under hypoxia. *Int. J. Biol. Sci.* 2010; 9;6(5):499-512.

[42] Horwitz EM, M Dominici. How do mesenchymal stromal cells exert their therapeutic benefit? *Cytotherapy* 2008; 10:771–774.

[43] Guillot PV, C Gotherstrom, J Chan, H Kurata and NM Fisk. Human first-trimester fetal MSC express Pluripotency markers and grow faster and have longer telomeres than adult MSC. *Stem Cells* 2007; 25:646–654.

[44] Pal R, Gopinath C, Rao NM, Banerjee P, Krishnamoorthy V, Venkataramana NK, Totey S. Functional recovery after transplantation of bone marrow-derived human mesenchymal stromal cells in a rat model of spinal cord injury. *Cytotherapy.* 2010; 12(6):792-806.

[45] Sotiropoulou PA, Perez SA, Salagianni M, Baxevanis CN, Papamichail M. Characterization of the optimal culture conditions for clinical scale production of human mesenchymal stem cells. Stem Cells. 2006; 24 (2):462-71.

[46] Govindasamy V, Ronald VS, Totey S, Din SB, Mustafa WM, Totey S, Zakaria Z, Bhonde RR. Micromanipulation of culture niche permits long-term expansion of dental pulp stem cells--an economic and commercial angle. In Vitro *Cell Dev. Biol. Anim.* 2010;46(9):764-73.

[47] Haynesworth SE, Goshima J, Goldberg VM, Caplan AI. Characterization of cells with osteogenic potential from human marrow. *Bone*. 1992; 13(1):81-8.

[48] Mauney J, Volloch V, Kaplan DL. Role of adult mesenchymal stem cells in bone tissue engineering applications. Current status and future prospects. *Tissue Eng*. 2005; 11: 787-802.

[49] Gimble J, Guilak F. Adipose-derived adult stem cells: isolation, characterization, and differentiation potential. *Cytotherapy*. 2003; 5(5):362-9.

[50] Mathews S, Bhonde R, Gupat PK, Totey S. Extracellular matrix protein mediated regulation of the osteoblast differentiation of bone marrow derived human mesenchymal stem cells. Differentiation 2012; 84(2):185-92. Epub. 2012 Jun 2.

[51] Govindasamy V, Abdullah AN, Ronald VS, Musa S, Ab Aziz ZA, Zain RB, Totey S, Bhonde RR, Abu Kasim NH. Inherent differential propensity of dental pulp stem cells derived from human deciduous and permanent teeth. *J. Endod.* 2010; 36(9):1504-15.

[52] Lian JB, Stein GS. Concepts of osteoblast growth and differentiation: basis for modulation of bone cell development and tissue formation. *Crit. Rev. Oral Biol. Med.* 1992; 3(3):269-305.

[53] Pockwinse SM, Wilming LG, Conlon DM, Stein GS, Lian JB. Expression of cell growth and bone specific genes at single cell resolution during development of bone tissue-like organization in primary osteoblast cultures. *J. Cell Biochem.* 1992; 49(3):310-23.

[54] Tsiridis E, Upadhyay N, Giannoudis P. Molecular aspects of fracture healing: which are the important molecules? *Injury*. 2007; 38 Suppl 1:S11-25.

[55] Dimitriou R, Tsiridis E, Giannoudis PV. Current concepts of molecular aspects of bone healing. *Injury* 2005; 36(12):1392-404.

[56] Dimitriou R, Jones E, McGonagle D, Giannoudis PV. Bone regeneration: current concepts and future directions. *BMC Med*. 2011; 9:66.

[57] Gallea S, Lallemand F, Atfi A, Rawadi G, Ramez V, Spinella-Jaegle S, Kawai S, Faucheu C, Huet L, Baron R, Roman-Roman S.Activation of mitogen-activated protein kinase cascades is involved in regulation of bone morphogenetic protein-2-induced osteoblast differentiation in pluripotent C2C12 cells. *Bone* 2001, 28, 491.

[58] Jadlowiec JA, Celil AB, Hollinger JO.Bone tissue engineering: recent advances and promising therapeutic agents. *Expert Opin. Biol. Ther.* 2003; 3, 409-423.

[59] Yilgor P, Tuzlakoglu K, Reis RL, Hasirci N, Hasirci V. Incorporation of a sequential BMP-2/BMP-7 delivery system into chitosan-based scaffolds for bone tissue engineering. *Biomaterials*. 2009; 30(21):3551-9.

[60] Tang Y, Tang W, Lin Y, Long J, Wang H, Liu L, Tian W. Combination of bone tissue engineering and BMP-2 gene transfection promotes bone healing in osteoporotic rats. *Cell Biol. Int*. 2008; 32(9):1150-7.

[61] Guo X, Zheng Q, Kulbatski I, Yuan Q, Yang S, Shao Z, Wang H, Xiao B, Pan Z, Tang S. Bone regeneration with active angiogenesis by basic fibroblast growth factor gene transfected mesenchymal stem cells seeded on porous beta-TCP ceramic scaffolds. *Biomed. Mater.* 2006; 1(3):93-9.

[62] Qu D, Li J, Li Y, Gao Y, Zuo Y, Hsu Y, Hu J.ac Angiogenesis and osteogenesis enhanced by bFGF ex vivo gene therapy for bone tissue engineering in reconstruction of calvarial defects. *J. Biomed. Mater. Res.* A. 2011; 96(3):543-51.

[63] Chen G, Deng C, Li YP. TGF-β and BMP Signalling in Osteoblast Differentiation and Bone Formation. *Int. J. Biol. Sci.* 2012; 8:272-288.

[64] Tsiridis E, Pavlou G, Charity J, Tsiridis E, Gie G, West R. The safety and efficacy of bilateral simultaneous total hip replacement: an analysis of 2063 cases. *J. Bone Joint Surg. Br.* 2008 ; 90(8):1005-12.

[65] Keogh MB, O' Brien FJ, Daly JS. A novel collagen scaffold supports human osteogenesis--applications for bone tissue engineering. *Cell Tissue Res.* 2010; 340(1):169-77.

[66] Lieberman JR, Daluiski A, Einhorn TA. The role of growth factors in the repair of bone. Biology and clinical applications. *J. Bone Joint Surg. Am.* 2002; 84- A(6):1032-44.

[67] Maeda S, Hayashi M, Komiya S, Imamura T, Miyazono K (2004) Endogenous TGF-beta signaling suppresses maturation of osteoblastic mesenchymal cells. *Embo J.* 23: 552–563.

[68] Spinella-Jaegle S, Roman-Roman S, Faucheu C, Dunn FW, Kawai S, et al. (2001) Opposite effects of bone morphogenetic protein-2 and transforming growth factor-beta1 on osteoblast differentiation. *Bone* 29: 323–330.

[69] Alliston T, Choy L, Ducy P, Karsenty G, Derynck R (2001) TGF-beta-induced repression of CBFA1 by Smad3 decreases cbfa1 and osteocalcin expression and inhibits osteoblast differentiation. *Embo J.* 20: 2254–2272.

[70] Street J, Lenehan B.Vascular endothelial growth factor regulates osteoblast survival – evidence for an autocrine feedback mechanism. *J. Ortho. Surg. Res.* 2009; 4:19-32.

[71] Giustina A, Mazziotti G, Canalis E. Growth hormone, insulin-like growth factors, and the skeleton. *Endocr. Rev.* 2008; 29: 535–59.

[72] Sanchez-Fernandez MA, Gallois A, Riedl T, Jurdic P, Hoflack B. Osteoclasts control osteoblast chemotaxis via PDGF-BB/PDGF receptor beta signaling.*PLoS ONE.*2008; 3(10):e3537.

[73] Kirkham GR, Cartmell SH. Genes and. proteins involved in the regulation of osteogenesis. Topic in Tissue Engineering 2007; Eds N Ashammakhi, R Reis, E Chiellinivol 3: 1-22.

[74] Ducy P, Starbuck M, Priemel M, Shen J, Pinero G, Geoffroy V, Amling M, Karsenty G. A Cbfa1-dependent genetic pathway controls bone formation beyond embryonic development. *Genes. Dev.* 1999;13(8):1025-36.

[75] Sato M, Morii E, Komori T, Kawahata H, Sugimoto M, Terai K, Shimizu H, Yasui T, Ogihara H, Yasui N, Ochi T, Kitamura Y, Ito Y, Nomura S. Transcriptional regulation of osteopontin gene in vivo by PEBP2alpha A/CBFA1 and ETS1 in the skeletal tissue. *Oncogene.* 1998; 17: 1517-1525.

[76] Kern B, Shen J, Starbuck M, Karsenty G. Cbfa1contributes to the osteoblast specific expression of type-I collagen genes. *J. Biol. Chem.* 2001; 276: 7101-7107.

[77] Ducy P, Desbois C, Boyce B, Pinero G, Story B, Dunstan C, Smith E, Bonadio J, Goldstein S, Gundberg C, Bradley A, Karsenty G. Increased bone formation in osteocalcin-deficient mice. *Nature*. 1996; 382 (6590):448-52.

[78] Karsenty G. The central regulation of bone remodelling. *Trends Endocrinol. Metab.* 2000;11 (10):437-9.

[79] Zhang C. 2010; Transcriptional regulation of bone formation by the osteoblast-specific transcription factor Osx. *J. Orthop. Surg. Res.* 5: 37.

[80] Nakashima K, Zhou X, Kunkel G, Zhang Z, Deng JM, Behringer RR, de Crombrugghe B. The novel zinc finger-containing transcription factor osterix is required for osteoblast differentiation and bone formation. Cell. 2002; 108(1): 17-29.

[81] Tu Q, Valverde P, Chen J. 2006; Osterix enhances proliferation and osteogenic potential of bone marrow stromal cells. *Biochem. Biophys. Res. Commun.* 341(4): 1257-1265.

[82] Karin M, Liu Z, Zandi E. AP-1 function and regulation. *Curr. Opin. Cell Biol.* 1997; 9 (2):240-246.

[83] Wang ZQ, Ovitt C, Grigoriadis AE, Möhle-Steinlein U, Rüther U, Wagner EF. Bone and haematopoietic defects in mice lacking c-fos. *Nature*. 1992;360(6406):741-745.

[84] Simeone, A., Acampora, D., Pannese, M., D'Esposito, M., Stornaiuolo, A., Gulisano, M., Mallamaci, A., Kastury, K., Druck, T., Huebner, K. Boncinelli E. Cloning and characterization of two members of the vertebrate Dlx gene family. *Proc. Natl. Acad. Sci. U S A* 1994; 91:2250-4.

[85] Shirakabe K, Terasawa K, Miyama K, Shibuya H, Nishida E. *Genes. Cells* 2001; 6:851-6.

[86] Shirakabe K, Terasawa K, Miyama K, Shibuya H, Nishida E. Regulation of the activity of the transcription factor Runx2 by two homeobox proteins, Msx2 and Dlx5. *Genes. Cells*. 2001; 6(10):851-6.

[87] Ducy P. Cbfa1: a molecular switch in osteoblast biology. *Dev. Dyn.* 2000; 219(4):461-71.

[88] Ryoo HM, Hoffmann HM, Beumer T, Frenkel B, Towler DA, Stein GS, Stein JL, van Wijnen AJ, Lian JB. Stage-specific expression of Dlx-5 during osteoblast differentiation: involvement in regulation of osteocalcin gene expression *Mol. Endocrinol.* 1997; 11:1681-94.

[89] Hernandez EC, Mikos AG. New biomaterials as scaffolds for tissue engineering. *Pharm. Res.* 2008; 25: 2345-2347.

[90] Chen CC, Chueh JY, Tseng H, Huang HM, Lee SY. Preparation and characterization of biodegradable PLA polymeric blends. *Biomaterials* 2003; 24:1167-1173.

[91] Ma PX, Zhang R, Xiao G, Franceschi R. Engineering new bone tissue in vitro on highly porous poly(alpha-hydroxyl acids)/hydroxyapatite composite scaffolds. *J. Biomed. Mater. Res.* 2001; 54:284-93.

[92] Yang Y, Magnay JL, Cooling L, El HA. Development of a 'mechano-active' scaffold for tissue engineering. *Biomaterials* 2002; 23:2119-26.

[93] Zhang R, Ma PX. Poly(alpha-hydroxyl acids)/hydroxyapatite porous composites for bone tissue engineering. I. Preparation and morphology. *J. Biomed. Mater. Res.* 1999; 44: 446-455.

[94] Andriano KP, Tabata Y, Ikada Y, Heller J. In vitro and in vivo comparison of bulk and surface hydrolysis in absorbable polymer scaffolds for tissue engineering. *J. Biomed. Mater. Res.* 1999; 48:602-12.

[95] Karp JM, Shoichet MS, Davies JE. Bone formation on two-dimensional poly(DL-lactide-coglycolide) (PLGA) films and three-dimensional PLGA tissue engineering scaffolds in vitro. *J. Biomed. Mater. Res.* 2003; 64A:388-96.

[96] Marra KG, Szem JW, Kumta PN, DiMilla PA, Weiss LE. In vitro analysis of biodegradable polymer blend/hydroxyapatite composites for bone tissue engineering. *J. Biomed. Mater. Res.* 1999; 47:324-35.

[97] Behravesh E, Yasko AW, Engel PS, Mikos AG. Synthetic biodegradable polymers for orthopaedic applications. *Clin. Orthop.* 1999; S118-29.

[98] Cooke MN, Fisher JP, Dean D, Rimnac C, Mikos AG. Use of stereolithography to manufacture critical-sized 3D biodegradable scaffolds for bone ingrowth. *J. Biomed. Mater. Res.* 2003; 64B:65-9.

[99] Brunski JB. Metals. In: Ratner, B.D., Hoffman, A.S., Schoen, F.J., et al., eds. Biomaterials Science: An Introduction to Materials in Medicine. New York: Academic Press, 1996, pp. 37–50.

[100] Hench LL. Ceramics, glasses, and glass-ceramics. In: Ratner, B.D., Hoffman, A.S., Schoen, F.J., et al., eds. Biomaterials Science: An Introduction to Materials in Medicine. New York: Academic Press, 1996, pp. 73–83.

[101] Allori AC, Sailon AM, Warren SM. Biological basis of bone formation, remodeling, and repair-part II: extracellular matrix. Tissue *Eng. Part B Rev.* 2008; 14(3):275-83.

[102] Hidalgo-Bastida LA, Cartmell SH. Mesenchymal stem cells, osteoblasts and extracellular matrix proteins: enhancing cell adhesion and differentiation for bone tissue engineering. *Tissue Eng. Part B Rev.* 2010; 4: 405-412.

[103] Mizuno M, Kuboki Y. Osteoblast-related gene expression of bone marrow cells during the osteoblastic differentiation induced by type I collagen, *J. Biochem.* 2001; 129: 133–138.

[104] Chevallay B, Herbage D. Collagen-based biomaterials as 3D scaffold for cell cultures: applications for tissue engineering and gene therapy. *Med. Biol. Eng. Comput.* 2000; 38(2):211-8.

[105] Munisamy S, Vaidyanathan TK, Vaidyanathan J. A bone-like precoating strategy for implants: collagen immobilization and mineralization on pure titanium implant surface. *J. Oral Implantol.* 2008; 34: 67-75.

[106] Zhang YZ, Su B, Venugopal J, Ramakrishna S, Lim CT. Biomimetic and bioactive nanofibrous scaffolds from electrospun composite nanofibers. *Int. J. Nanomedicine.* 2007; 2(4):623-38.

[107] Hattar S, Asselin A, Greenspan D, Oboeuf M, Berdal A, Sautier JM. Potential of biomimetic surfaces to promote in vitro osteoblast-like cell differentiation. *Biomaterials.* 2005; 26(8):839-48.

[108] Vagaská B, Bacáková L, Filová E, Balík K. Osteogenic cells on bio-inspired materials for bone tissue engineering. *Physiol. Res.* 2010;59(3):309-22.

[109] Semino CE. Self-assembling peptides: from bio-inspired materials to bone regeneration. *J. Dent. Res.* 2008 Jul;87(7):606-16.

[110] Hoshiba T, Kawazoe N, Chen G. Mechanism of regulation of PPARG expression of mesenchymal stem cells by osteogenesis-mimicking extracellular matrices.Biosci. *Biotechnol. Biochem.* 2011;75(11):2099-104.

[111] Sasano Y, Li HC, Zhu JX, Imanaka-Yoshida K, Mizoguchi I, Kagayama M. Immunohistochemical localization of type I collagen, fibronectin and tenascin C during embryonic osteogenesis in the dentary of mandibles and tibias in rats. *Histochem J.* 2000; 32(10):591-8.

[112] Kamiya N, Shigemasa K, Takagi M. Gene expression and immunohistochemical localization of decorin and biglycan in association with early bone formation in the developing mandible. *J. Oral Sci.* 2001;43(3):179-88.

[113] Rodan GA, Noda M. Gene expression in osteoblastic cells. *Crit. Rev. Eukaryot. Gene. Expr.* 1991;1 (2):85-98.

[114] Gong Z, Wezeman FH. Inhibitory effect of alcohol on osteogenic differentiation in human bone marrow-derived mesenchymal stem cells. *Alcohol Clin. Exp Res.* 2004; 28(3): 468-479.

[115] Ducy P, Zhang R, Geoffroy V, Ridall AL, Karsenty G. Osf2/Cbfa1: a transcriptional activator of osteoblast differentiation. *Cell.* 1997 May 30;89(5):747-54.

[116] Komori T. Regulation of osteoblast differentiation by Runx2. *Adv. Exp. Med. Biol.* 2010; 658: 43-49.

[117] Kundu AK, Putnam AJ. Vitronectin and collagen I differentially regulate osteogenesis in mesenchymal stem cells. *Biochem. Biophys. Res. Commun.* 2006; 347: 347-357.

[118] Salasznyk RM, Williams WA, Boskey A, Batorsky A, Plopper GE. Adhesion to vitronectin and collagen promotes osteogenic differentiation of human mesenchymal stem cells. *J. Biomed. Biotech.* 2004; 2004(1):24-34.

[119] Wight TN, Kinsella MG, Eva EQ. The role of proteoglycans in cell adhesion, migration and proliferation. *Curr. Opin. Cell Biol.* 1992; 4(5): 793-780.

[120] Ashhurst DE, Ashton BA, Owen ME. The collagens and glycosaminoglycans of the extracellular matrices secreted by bone marrow stromal cells cultured in vivo in diffusion chambers. *J. Orthop. Res.* 1990;8(5): 741-749.

[121] Gallagher JT, Spooncer E, Dexter TM. Role of the cellular matrix in haemopoiesis: I. Synthesis of glycosaminoglycans by mouse bone marrow cell cultures. *J. Cell Sci.* 1983; 63: 155-171.

[122] Siczkowski M, Andrew T, Amos S, Gordon MY. Hyaluronic acid regulates the function and distribution of sulfated glycosaminoglycans in bone marrow stromal cultures. *Exp. Hematol.* 1993; 21(1): 126-30.

[123] Kazama T, Takagi M, Ishii T, Toda Y. Immunoelectron microscopic studies glycosaminoglycans in the metaphyseal bone trabeculae of growing rats. *Histochemical J.* 1992; 24(10): 747-755.

[124] Taipale J, Keski-Oja J. Growth factors in the extracellular matrix. *FASEB J.* 1997; 11: 51-59.

[125] Benoit DS, Anseth KS. Heparin functionalized PEG gels that modulate protein adsorption for hMSC adhesion and differentiation. *Acta. Biomater.* 2005; 1(4): 461-70.

[126] Sun Y, Li W, Lu Z, Chen R, Ling J, Ran Q, Jilka RL, Chen XD. Rescuing replication and osteogenesis of aged mesenchymal stem cells by exposure to a young extracellular matrix. *FASEB J.* 2011; 25(5): 1474-1485.

[127] Wollenweber M, Domaschke H, Hanke T, Boxberger S, Schmack G, Gliesche K, Scharnweber D, Worch H. Mimicked bioartificial matrix containing chondroitin sulphate on a textile scaffold of poly(3-hydroxybutyrate) alters the differentiation of adult human mesenchymal stem cells. *Tissue Eng.* 2006; 12(2): 345-359.
[128] Lian JB, Stein GS. Development of the osteoblast phenotype: molecular mechanisms mediating osteoblast growth and differentiation. *Iowa Orthop. J.* 1995; 15: 118-140.
[129] Lian JB, Stein JL, Stein GS, van Wijnen AJ, Montecino M, Javed A, Gutierrez S, Shen J, Zaidi SK, Drissi H. Runx2/Cbfa1 functions: diverse regulation of gene transcription by chromatin remodeling and co-regulatory protein interactions. *Connect Tissue Res.* 2003;44Suppl 1:141-8.
[130] Kim J, Kim IS, Cho TH, Lee KB, Hwang SJ, Tae G, Noh I, Lee SH, Park Y, Sun K. Bone regeneration using hyaluronic acid-based hydrogel with bone morphogenic protein-2 and human mesenchymal stem cells. *Biomaterials.* 2007; 28(10): 1830-1837.
[131] Manferdini C, Guarino V, Zini N, Raucci MG, Ferrari A, Grassi F, Gabusi E, Squarzoni S, Facchini A, Ambrosio L, Lisignoli G. Mineralization behavior with mesenchymal stromal cells in a biomimetic hyaluronic acid-based scaffold. *Biomaterials.* 2010; 31(14): 3986-3996.
[132] Huang L, Cheng YY, Koo PL, Lee KM, Qin L, Cheng JC, Kumta SM. The effect of hyaluronan on osteoblast proliferation and differentiation in rat calvarial derived cell cultures. *J. Biomed. Mater. Res. A.* 2003; 66(4): 880-884.
[133] Kawano M, Ariyoshi W, Iwanaga K, Okinaga T, Habu M, Yoshioka I, Tominaga K, Nishihara T. Mechanism involved in enhancement of osteoblast differentiation by hyaluronic acid. *Biochem. Biophys. Res. Commun.* 2011; 405(4): 575-580.
[134] Jha AK, Xu X, Duncan RL, Jia X. Controlling the adhesion and differentiation of mesenchymal stem cells using hyaluronic acid-based, doubly cross-linked networks. *Biomaterials.* 2011; 32(10): 2466-2478.
[135] Underhill C. CD44: the hyaluronan receptor. *J. Cell Sci.* 1992; 103(2): 293-298.
[136] Peterson RS, Andhare RA, Rousche KT, Knudson W, Wang W, Grossfield JB, Thomas RO, Hollingsworth RE, Knudson CB. CD44 modulates Smad1 activation in the BMP-7 signalling pathway. *J. Cell Biol.* 2004; 166(7): 1081-1091.
[137] Ma PX. Biomimetic Materials for Tissue Engineering. *Adv. Drug. Deliv. Rev.* 2008; 60(2): 184–198.
[138] Ripamonti U, Roden L. Biomimetics for the induction of bone formation. *Expert Rev. Med. Devices.* 2010; 7(4):469-79.
[139] Zhang Y, Reddy VJ, Wong SY, Li X, Su B, Ramakrishna S, Lim CT. Enhanced biomineralization in osteoblasts on a novel electrospunbiocompositenanofibrous substrate of hydroxyapatite /collagen/chitosan. *Tissue Eng. Part A.* 2010; 16(6):1949-60.
[140] Nair LS, Laurencin CT. Polymers as biomaterials for tissue engineering and controlled drug delivery. *Adv. Biochem. Eng. Biotechnol.* 2006; 102: 47-90.
[141] Peniche C, Fernández M, Rodríguez G, Parra J, Jimenez J, Bravo AL, Gómez D, San Román J. Cell supports of chitosan/hyaluronic acid and chondroitin sulphate systems. Morphology and biological behaviour. *J. Mater. Sci. Mater. Med.* 2007; 18(9): 1719-1726.

[142] Yang X, Chen X, Wang H. Acceleration of osteogenic differentiation of preosteoblastic cells by chitosan containing nanofibrous scaffolds. *Biomacromolecules*. 2009; 10(10): 2772-2778.

[143] Venkatesan J, Kim SK. Chitosan composites for bone tissue engineering—an overview. *Mar. Drugs*. 2010; 8(8): 2252-2266.

[144] Francesko A, Tzanov T. Chitin, chitosan and derivatives for wound healing and tissue engineering. *Adv. Biochem. Eng. Biotechnol.* 2011; 125:1-27.

[145] Manjubala I, Ponomarev I, Wilke I, Jandt KD. Growth of osteoblast-like cells on biomimetic apatite-coated chitosan scaffolds. *J. Biomed. Mater. Res B Appl. Biomater.* 2008; 84(1):7-16.

[146] Mathews S, Gupta PK, Bhonde R, Totey S. Chitosan enhances mineralization during osteoblast differentiation of human bone marrow-derived mesenchymal stem cells, by upregulating the associated genes. *Cell Prolif.* 2011; 44: 537-549.

[147] Clegg RE, Leavesley DI, Pearcy MJ. Mediation of biomaterial–cell interactions by adsorbed proteins: *A Review. Tissue Eng*. 2005; 11: 1-18.

[148] Zhang C. Transcriptional regulation of bone formation by the osteoblast-specific transcription factor *Osx. J. Orthop. Surg. Res*. 2010; 5: 37.

[149] Kulterer B, Friedl G, Jandrositz A, Sanchez-Cabo F, Prokesch A, Paar C, Scheideler M, Windhager R, Preisegger KH, Trajanoski Z. Gene expression profiling of human mesenchymal stem cells derived from bone marrow during expansion and osteoblast differentiation. *BMC Genomics*. 2007; 8: 70-55.

[150] Karner E, Unger C, Sloan AJ, Richter LA, Sugars RV, Wendel M. Bone matrix formation in osteogenesis cultures derived from human embryonic stem cells in vitro. *Stem Cells Dev*. 2007; 16: 1-13.

[151] Rafat M, Li F, Fagerholm P, Lagali NS, Watsky MA, Munger R, Matsuura T, Griffith M. PEG-stabilized carbodiimidecrosslinked collagen-chitosan hydrogels for corneal tissue engineering. *Biomaterials*. 2008; 29: 3960-3972.

[152] Wang XH, Li DP, Wang WJ, Feng QL, Cui FZ, Xu YX, Song XH, van der Werf M. Crosslinked collagen/chitosan matrix for artificial livers, *Biomaterials*. 2003; 24: 3213-3220.

[153] Mathews S, Bhonde R, Gupta PK, Totey S. A novel tripolymer coating demonstrating the synergistic effect of chitosan, collagen type 1 and hyaluronic acid on osteogenic differentiation of human bone marrow derived mesenchymal stem cells. *Biochem. Biophys. Res. Communic*. 2011; 414: 270-276.

[154] Ma L, Gao C, Mao Z, Zhou J, Shen J, Hu X, Han C. Collagen/chitosan porous scaffolds with improved biostability for skin tissue engineering. *Biomaterials*. 2003; 24(26):4833-41.

[155] Di Martino A, Sittinger M, Risbud MV. Chitosan: a versatile biopolymer for orthopaedic tissue-engineering. *Biomaterials*. 2005; 26(30):5983-90.

[156] Huang Y, Onyeri S, Siewe M, Moshfeghian A, Madihally SV. In vitro characterization of chitosan-gelatin scaffolds for tissue engineering. *Biomaterials*. 2005; 26(36):7616-27.

[157] Jana S, Florczyk SJ, Leung M, Zhang M. High-strength pristine porous chitosan scaffolds for tissue engineering. *J. Mater. Chem*. 2012; 22: 6291-6299.

[158] Austin K. Scaffold design: use of chitosan in cartilage tissue engineering. *Basic Biotechnology eJournal*. 2007; 3:62-66.

[159] J.M Oliveira, M.T Rodrigues, S.S Silva, P.B Malafaya, M.E Gomes, C.A Viegas, I.R Dias, J.T Azevedo, J.F Mano and R.L Reis: Novel hydroxyapatite/chitosan bilayered scaffold for osteochondral tissue engineering applications: Scaffold Design and its performance when seeded with goat bone marrow stromal cells. *Biomaterials* 2006, 276:123-6137.
[160] Globus RK, Doty SB, Lull JC, Holmuhamedov E, Humphries MJ, Damsky CH. Fibronectin is a survival factor for differentiated osteoblasts. *J. Cell Sci.* 1998; 111 (pt 10):1385-93.
[161] Kalfas IH. Principles of bone healing. *Neurosurg Focus.* 2001; 10: 7-10.
[162] Morra M. Biochemical modification of titanium surfaces: peptides and ECM proteins. *Eur. Cell Mater.* 2006; 12: 1-15.
[163] Rammelt S, Schulze E, Bernhardt R, Hanisch U, Scharnweber D, Worch H, Zwipp H, Biewener A. Coating of titanium implants with type-I collagen. *J. Orthop. Res.* 2004; 22: 1025-1034.

In: Osteoblasts
Editor: Hugo Scheurer
ISBN: 978-1-62417-806-1

Chapter 3

Osteoblast Functions and their Role in Skeletal Bone Diseases

Eman Allam, Pierre Eleniste, Angela Bruzzaniti and L. Jack Windsor *

Department of Oral Biology, Indiana University School of Dentistry, Indianapolis, IN, US

Abstract

Osteoblasts are highly specialized mesenchymal cells that are responsible for the formation and maintenance of the skeletal architecture. They produce extracellular matrix proteins and are regulators of matrix mineralization during bone formation and remodeling. Osteoblasts regulate the activity of osteoclasts through the secretion of cytokines such as receptor activator of nuclear factor κ-B ligand, macrophage colony stimulating factor and osteoprotegerin. In many pathological conditions, bone formation and remodeling are dysregulated and osteoblasts have a major role in the pathogenesis of these disorders. Abnormalities in the differentiation and functions of osteoblasts occur in several common human diseases such as osteoporosis and osteoarthritis. In late-stage osteoporosis, osteoblasts exhibit decreased proliferation rates and abnormal functions, while in osteoarthritis abnormal behaviors and metabolism are observed. There are also some rare human diseases, such as van Buchem's disease, in which osteoblast activity is increased leading to a high bone mass phenotype. In addition, some solid tumors metastasize to the skeleton as a result of dysregulated osteoblast activity. This chapter will summarize the current knowledge about osteoblast functions and their role in skeletal bone diseases.

* Corresponding author/contact author - L. Jack Windsor, Ph.D. Indiana University School of Dentistry, Department of Oral Biology, 1121 W. Michigan Street, Room 271, Indianapolis, Indiana 46202; Associate Professor of Oral Biology, School of Dentistry, Adjunct Associate Professor of Anatomy and Cell Biology, School of Medicine, Director, Tobacco Cessation and Biobehavioral Group; PHONE: (317) 274-1448; FAX: (317) 278-1411; E-MAIL: ljwindso@iupui.edu.

Introduction

Bone is continuously remodeled through the actions of bone cells and an imbalance in this process can result in various bone diseases. There are three major bone cells: osteoclasts, osteoblasts, and osteocytes. Osteoclasts are responsible for bone resorption, while osteoblasts are responsible for new bone formation. Osteocytes are terminally differentiated osteoblasts that become entrapped within the matrix and play important roles in sensing mechanical strains and bone damage [1-6].

In addition to their roles in regulating bone matrix production and mineralization, osteoblasts also play a significant role in controlling bone resorption through the expression of nuclear factor-kB (RANK) ligand (RANKL) and secretion of osteoprotegerin (OPG) [7]. In addition to bone formation, osteoblasts secrete proteins, such as FoxO1, with autocrine, paracrine, and endocrine functions which regulate cellular processes beyond bone formation [8, 9]. Therefore, osteoblasts have multi-functional roles in regulating bone homeostasis. In this review, the current knowledge of osteoblast biology and its implications in various bone diseases will be summarized and discussed.

Osteoblast Lineage and Differentiation

Selective transcriptional regulators of mesenchymal stem cells (MSCs) give rise to a variety of cells including fibroblasts, chondrocytes, myoblasts, adipocytes and osteoblasts [10-16]. Osteoblast differentiation from MSCs follows a multi-step process. Mesenchymal progenitors give rise to preosteoblasts, osteoblasts, bone-lining cells and osteocytes [17-19]. During differentiation, osteoblasts secrete extracellular matrix components such as type I collagen and fibronectin, as well as signaling molecules such as transforming growth factor (TGF-β), and subsequently differentiate into mature osteoblasts. The mature osteoblasts are then responsible for the matrix mineralization process [20]. During this complicated process, some osteoblasts become embedded into the newly formed bone matrix and become osteocytes. The remaining mature osteoblasts either die or become quiescent bone-lining cells.

Transcription Factors, Signaling Proteins and Osteoblast Differentiation

Osteoblast differentiation and activity are influenced by the expression of various transcription factors, hormones, and signaling proteins (Table 1) [21-33]. For example, two of the most widely studied osteoblast transcription factors are Runx2 and osterix (also known as SP7) [15,16,22]. The Runx family is composed of three genes: Runx1, Runx2 and Runx3. Runx2 is critical for osteoblast differentiation and chondrocyte hypertrophy [34,35]. In contrast, Runx1 is essential for hematopoietic stem cell differentiation [36,37], while Runx3 play roles in neurogenesis and regulates growth of gastric epithelial cells [38]. As mentioned, Runx2 is critically involved during osteoblastogenesis through up-regulation of various osteoblast genes such as type I collagen, osteopontin, bone sialoprotein and osteocalcin [15, 39-41]. Runx-2-deficient mice lack bone tissue due to the absence of osteoblasts [15,16]. Recent studies have demonstrated that Runx2 expression is also a key pathological factor in osteosarcomas by regulating cancer-related genes [42,43] and cell proliferation [44]. Since Runx2 is crucial for bone formation, the challenge is finding ways to regulate Runx2 expression in osteosarcoma cells while avoiding suppression of bone growth. Osterix (Osx) is a zinc finger transcription factor that is important for osteoblast differentiation, bone formation and mineralization [45]. Studies in mice with a targeted deletion of Osx provided insights into the physiological relevance of Osx for bone formation. Nakashima and colleagues showed that cartilage was formed as normal in Osx-null embryos, but the embryos lacked bone formation [45]. They also observed that cells in the periosteum and in the condensed mesenchyme of membranous skeletal elements cannot differentiate into osteoblasts. However, these cells do express Runx2. Unexpectedly, they also reported that Osx was not expressed in Runx2-null mice, suggesting that Osx acts downstream of Runx2. This was experimentally confirmed by Nishio and colleagues, who demonstrated a direct link between Runx2 and Osx gene transcription [28].

Table 1. Key signaling proteins in osteoblasts

Protein	Role	Ref
Runx2	Induces osteoblast differentiation and bone formation. Deletion of Runx2 lead to systemic bone loss.	[38, 45]
β-catenin	Conditional deletion of the β-catenin gene in osteoblasts in vivo leads to reduced bone mass.	[143-146]
Osterix	Essential for differentiation of preosteoblasts into mature osteoblasts.	[147-148]
Twist	Interacts with Runx2 and inhibits Runx2 function during osteoblast differentiation without affecting Runx2 expression.	[30]
AFT4	Critical regulator of OB differentiation and function. Deletion of AFT4 leads to severe skeletal defects.	[145, 149]
SMADS	Smad1 KO causes calvarial bone development delay. Smad4 KO leads to lower bone mineral density, decreased bone volume, decreased bone formation rate and osteoblast numbers. Smad7 inhibits chondrocyte differentiation at multiple steps during endochondral bone formation.	[52,150-152]
Shn3	Plays an important role in regulating skeletal development and OB differentiation.	[32]
Dlx5	Dlx5-deficient mice showed defects in bone formation. Dlx5 also upregulates expression of alkaline phosphatase and osteocalcin.	[29,153-155]
BMPS	BMP2 leads to spontaneous fractures BMP2/BMP4 KO leads to severe impairment of osteogenesis and to a severe chondrodysplasia phenotype.	[156-157]
TGF-β	TGF-β favors osteoblast proliferation but restricts osteoblast maturation, mainly by repressing the expression of genes involved in bone formation.	[158]

Activating transcription factor 4 (ATF4) is known to be essential for proliferation and differentiation of osteoblasts. Various studies have demonstrated that deletion of Atf4 in mice caused delay of bone formation during embryonic development and the mice displayed low bone mass throughout postnatal life. [25, 33, 46]. Yang and colleagues reported that ATF4 forms a complex with Runx2 and this cooperative interaction stimulates osteoblast-specific osteocalcin (Ocn) expression [47]. Recently, it has been shown that ATF4 is also required for parathyroid hormone (PTH) induction of Ocn expression in osteoblasts [48,49].

The Smad proteins are a small family of eukaryotic transcription regulators that play key roles in the transforming growth factor-beta signaling cascade [50]. It has been shown that the loss of Smad3 results in a lower rate of bone formation and osteopenia in addition to defects in chondrocyte differentiation [51]. Others showed that Smad4 mutant mice have lower bone mass and that Smad4 is required for the normal organization of the cartilage growth plate. This was further validated by studies showing that bone mineral density, bone volume, bone formation rate, and osteoblast numbers and function were dramatically reduced in Smad4 mutant mice [52].

Osteoblast Migration

Integrins are a large family of heterodimeric transmembrane glycoproteins that bind to extracellular matrix ligands, cell-surface ligands, and soluble ligands. Each integrin is a heterodimer consisting of an independent α subunit and β subunit [53-55]. Osteoblasts have been shown to express a wide variety of integrins including integrin αvβ3, αvβ5, αvβ1, α2β1, α4β1, and α5β1, as well as bone matrix proteins (e.g., osteopontin, bone sialoprotein (BSP), vitronectin, collagen, and fibronectin) [1, 56-59]. It is well-established that integrin-mediated adhesion of cells to extracellular matrix components is essential for cell migration, proliferation, survival, and differentiation [53, 60]. The importance of the matrix-integrin interactions on osteoblast function was demonstrated when osteoblasts were cultured on BSP, collagen, or osteopontin, which altered the proliferation and differentiation profile of the osteoblasts [61-63].

Osteoblast migration is an important step in modeling, remodeling, and fracture healing. Various chemical inhibitors have profound effects on osteoblast migration. For example, Felix and colleagues demonstrated that bisphosphonates disturbed osteoblast morphology and migration. They attributed this event to the influence of bisphosphonates on increasing integrin αvβ3 and tenascin C gene expression, both of which are crucial for cell shape and focal adhesion [64].

Dynamin is a mechanochemical GTPase that has been shown to participate in several cellular functions including clathrin-mediated endocytosis, caveolae-mediated internalization, and actin cytoskeletal remodeling [65-70]. In osteoclasts and other highly migratory cells, dynamin acts in a GTPase-dependent manner to promote the disassembly of actin in podosomes [71, 72] and decreases the phosphorylation of Pyk2, a focal adhesion protein [73, 74]. It has also been reported that dynamin regulates the bone resorbing activity and migration of osteoclasts [72]. However, the role of dynamin in osteoblast activity still remains unclear. Using primary calvaria-derived osteoblasts, we found that multiple isoforms of dynamin are expressed in osteoblasts. In addition, a chemical inhibitor of dynamin GTPase activity lead to an increase in the number of focal adhesions and a decrease in osteoblast migration (55 and unpublished data). These findings suggest dynamin's GTPase activity is important for regulating osteoblast migration.

Osteoblasts and Bone Diseases

Osteoporosis

Osteoporosis is a disorder of reduced bone mineral density and alteration of bone microarchitecture resulting in increased risks of fractures. The disease is attributable to the pathological loss of the balance between bone resorption by osteoclasts and bone formation by osteoblasts, resulting in alteration in the remodeling process [75, 76]. While postmenopausal osteoporosis is due to an increased bone resorbing activity of osteoclasts caused by estrogen deficiency, osteoporosis in later stages of life also involves defective osteoblastic functions [77]. The change in the rate of bone turnover with age is responsible for net bone loss. The number and activity of osteoblasts are decreased resulting in reduced osteoblastic bone formation compared to osteoclastic bone resorption. At the tissue level, the impaired osteoblastic bone formation with age translates into reduced cortical thickness and decreased newly formed trabecular bone [77, 78]. The age-related osteoblast dysfunction is due to both external and internal factors. External factors are mediated by age-related changes in the bone microenvironment such as changes in the levels of hormones and growth factors, while the internal factors are primarily caused by osteoblast cellular senescence. As a result, both trabecular and periosteal bone formation decrease with age in both genders. In senile osteoporosis, this age-related progressive bone loss is exaggerated resulting in decreased bone mass, increased bone fragility, and increased risks of fractures. Interestingly, external factors also affect bone loss. Smoking and use of alcohol are two major contributing risk factors for osteoporosis and increased fracture risk. Reports indicate that the risk is mediated through the direct inhibitory actions of these agents, or their byproducts, on osteoblast proliferation and differentiation, thus adversely affecting bone metabolism and reducing bone density [79-82]. The proliferation of MG63, an osteoblast-like cell-line, was significantly reduced when cells were subjected to 1000 μg/ml of nicotine (Figure 1), which is equivalent to the concentration in the saliva of smokers. Although cytokine/growth factor expression by osteoblasts exposed to the same concentration of nicotine was not affected, zymography results showed that matrix metalloproteinase (MMP-2) expression was altered (unpublished data).

Osteoblasts from postmenopausal osteoporotic women are characterized by a lower proliferation rate and abnormal function compared to normal osteoblasts [83]. In vitro studies indicated that osteoblasts derived from patients with osteoporosis demonstrated increased tyrosine phosphorylation of the insulin-like growth factor (IGF-I) receptor together with reduced stimulation of receptor phosphorylation by the IGF-I receptor, suggesting that decreased bone formation in osteoporosis is correlated with the abnormalities of the IGF-I signaling system [84]. Compared to normal osteoblasts, osteoporotic osteoblasts revealed lower production of osteocalcin and a much lower response to 1,25 $(OH)_2$ Vitamin D3 [85]. Human osteoblasts isolated from osteoporotic patients also showed abnormal expression patterns of cytokines involved in the regulation of bone metabolism such as interleukin-6 (IL-

6) and TGF-β [86-87]. This indicated that osteoporotic osteoblasts possess a different metabolic phenotype that may be responsible in part on their reduced anabolic function.

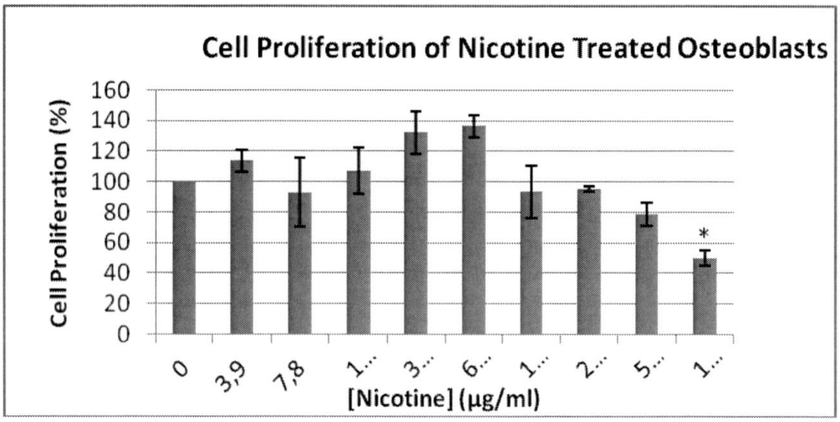

* denotes p=0.007.

Figure 1. Cell proliferation of MG63 cells at different concentrations of nicotine assessed by water-soluble tetrazolium-1 (WST-1) assay. A 1000 μg/ml concentration of nicotine reduced cellular proliferation by 49.9% compared to the control.

Studies on postmenopausal osteoporosis suggest that estrogen withdrawal affects osteoblast functions through the inhibition of pro-osteoblastic factors expressed by osteoclasts and that estrogen indirectly affects osteoblast-osteoclast coupling and the intercellular communication between the two cell types [78]. Reduced estrogen expression resulted in down regulation of several pro-osteoclast factors, such as IL-1, IL-6 and tumor necrosis factor (TNF), and also to the inhibition of OPG and stimulation of RANKL expression leading to an increase in osteoclast formation and bone resorption [88-91].

Wnt/β-catenin signaling in bone is one of the major pathways that control the process of bone formation. Activation of the Wnt/β-catenin pathway stimulates osteoblastic cell proliferation and differentiation. Genetic studies showed that LRP5/Wnt signaling pathway is anabolic for bone, promotes osteoblast survival, and interacts with bone morphogenetic protein-2 (BMP2) and parathyroid hormone (PTH), increasing osteoblastogenesis [92-96]. Studies in mice have also indicated that alterations in Wnt signaling contribute to age-related bone loss and that mechanical loading upregulates Wnt signaling in MSCs, suggesting that the combination of reduced β-catenin signaling and decreased mechanical stimulation contribute to age-related bone loss [97-98]. The critical role of Wnt signaling in bone formation provided the basis for several clinical trials. For example, activation of the Wnt signaling through the use of glycogen synthase kinase 3 inhibitors in ovariectomized mice resulted in increased bone formation and higher trabecular and cortical bone density and bone strength [99-100]. Increased bone anabolic markers in postmenopausal women together with increased bone formation in vivo in monkeys and ovariectomized rats after the systemic administration of inhibitors of Wnt antagonists have opened the door for a more promising approach to promote bone formation through the therapeutic use of inhibitors of Wnt signaling antagonists in clinical settings [101, 102]. An example of a Wnt antagonist that could be targeted to promote bone formation is DKK1. Studies showed that mice lacking DKK1 exhibited increased bone formation and bone mass while mice overexpressing DKK1 in osteoblasts were osteopenic [103, 104]. sFRP1 is another Wnt antagonist that acts by binding Wnt proteins and offers another promising treatment strategy. Studies in mice have shown that overexpression of sFRP1 inhibits in vivo bone formation, whereas deletion of sFRP1 increased bone mass [105].

As mentioned, OPG/RANK/RANKL is known to be the basic regulatory system for bone remodeling and it is also considered a main player in the pathogenesis of osteoporosis. OPG-deficient mice presented an osteoporotic phenotype and were accompanied by an increased rate of bone fractures. The up-regulation of RANKL in human bone marrow cells was shown to be a major determinant of increased bone resorption induced by estrogen deficiency [106-107]. A human monoclonal antibody against RANKL was very effective in reducing bone resorbing activity in postmenopausal women [108]. Many clinical trials have now confirmed the therapeutic potential of the RANKL antibody as a treatment for postmenopausal osteoporosis and in other skeletal diseases [77].

Osteoarthritis

Osteoarthritis (OA) is a chronic degenerative joint disease characterized by breakdown of cartilage. Changes in the cartilage and bones of the joint lead to pain, stiffness and use limitations. Several reports provided evidence for the involvement of subchondral bone in the progression and initiation of the cartilage degradation and the abnormal functions and metabolism of OA osteoblasts [109-111].

The subchondral bone sclerosis associated with OA is thought to play a key role in the progressive destruction of the cartilage observed in OA. The alterations in subchondral bone tissue microarchitecture and the excessive mineralization was suggested to be due to abnormal osteoblast metabolism [110]. Reports indicated that type I collagen levels are elevated in OA bone tissue compared to normal bone and that OA osteoblasts have increased collagen type I deposition, but with an altered ratio of collagen α1 and α2 chains, in particular with an increase of the α1 chain [112].

Comparison of the gene expression of normal bone and bone obtained from OA patients using microarray gene expression profiling has revealed differences in the expression of several genes that control osteoblast function and that are components of the Wnt and TGF-β/BMP signaling pathways. Furthermore, human osteoblasts derived from subchondral OA bone have been shown to express ephrin B2, which activates its receptor EphB4 and leads to inhibition of many resorption factors such as RANKL, IL-1β, and IL-6 [113-114].

Osteogenesis Imperfecta

Osteogenesis imperfecta (OI) is a disorder of congenital bone fragility. Patients suffer from bone deformities such as bowed legs or scoliosis, short stature, brittle teeth, muscle weakness, triangular face, hearing loss, and breathing problems. OA is caused mainly by mutations in 2 genes (*COL1A1* and *COL1A2)* that code for type I procollagen [115]. Specifically, genes that encode the polypeptide chains that make up the type I collagen triple helix, which is the major component of bone matrix. OI is considered a disease of osteoblast dysfunction, in which osteoblasts lay down an abnormal matrix that does not respond to mechanical loads. The osteoblast population increases and osteoclast activity is higher, leading to increased bone turnover rate [115].

Van Buchem Disease and Sclerosteosis

Van Buchem disease is a rare autosomal recessive sclerosing bone dysplasia that was first described by van Buchem et al. in 1955. The condition was first called "hyperostosis corticalis generalisata familiaris," and was characterized by increased cortical bone thickness and density affecting the skull, mandible, and shafts of the long bones. Clinically, the patient suffers macrocephaly and remarkably enlarged mandible which can be very broad and prognatic. This characteristic endosteal hyperostosis or hyperstotic bone of the skull and the mandible may lead in some cases to neurologic pain, hearing or visual problems, headaches and facial nerve palsy [116-117]. Van Buchem is caused by mutation in SOST gene that code for sclerostin, which is responsible on inhibiting bone formation. The newly formed bone is qualitatively normal with normal mineral content, but is associated with elevated alkaline phosphatase in serum [116-117].

Sclerosteosis is a bone disease caused by loss of function of SOST (sclerostin) and is characterized by high bone mass due to increased osteoblast activity. The data from the study by Brunkow and colleague demonstrated that the majority of the affected individuals have been reported in the Afrikaner population of South Africa, where a high incidence of the disorder occurs. To understand the molecular mechanisms, Sutherland and colleagues using null SOST mutation mouse as a model of the sclerosteosis, showed that BMPs-2, 4, and 6 induced an increased in the levels of SOST in a time- and dose-dependent manner. BMP's stimulatory effects on SOST were further enhanced by retinoic acid or 1,25-dihydroxyvitamin D3. They postulated that the levels of SOST expression are potentially modulated by BMPs [118,119].

Oculodentodigital Dysplasia

Dysfunctional osteoblasts have been linked to oculodentodigital dysplasia (ODDD) [120-122]. ODDD is characterized by craniofacial bone deformities and limb abnormalities. Connexin 43 (Cx43)-null mice are considered a model for ODDD. Osteoblasts from these mice exhibit abnormal differentiation and delayed mineralization and ossification [120, 123-125]. Therefore, Cx43 plays an important role in osteoblastic differentiation in vitro and bone formation in vivo [126].

Camurati-Engelmann Disease

Camurati-Engelmann disease is characterized by bone pain, which is caused by mutations in TGF-β1. It is known that TGF-β1 affects both osteoblasts and osteoclasts, and acts as a coupling factor between bone deposition and resorption [118]. Recently, a new TGF-β1 mutation (E169K) in exon 2 was identified in a Chinese family [127]. This mutation has not been previously reported in other countries in the world. However, the molecular mechanisms by which TGF-β1 or other important signaling proteins leads to Camurati-Engelmann disease is not yet clear.

Cleidocranial Dysplaysia

As mentioned previously, Runx2 is an essential transcription factor required for skeletal development and cartilage formation. Haploinsufficiency of Runx2 leads to cleidocranial displaysia (CCD), a bone disorder characterized by gross dysgenesis of bones mainly those derived from intramembranous bone formation. In their studies, Piero and colleagues looked at the effects of strontium on gene expression of bone marker proteins, the formation of hydroxyapatite and the cell proliferation of strontium-treated Runx2+/− osteoblasts. Their data showed that strontium improved matrix mineralization of mature Runx2+/− osteoblasts mainly by activation of cell proliferation [128]. Unlike normal osteoblasts, gene expression of bone marker proteins was not affected in strontium-treated Runx2+/− osteoblasts, while improved hydroxyapatite formation was noted in the extracellular matrix.

Osteoblastic Bone Metastasis

Bone metastasis and other malignancy associated skeletal complications such as hypercalcemia, bone pain, and pathological fractures are caused by disruption of the balanced regulation of the processes of bone formation that is mediated by osteoblasts and bone resorption that is mediated by osteoclasts. This balanced process of bone remodeling becomes disturbed by tumor cells and this dramatically accelerates bone remodeling resulting in a spectrum of osteolytic to osteoblastic bone lesions. The characterization of bone metastases as either osteoblastic or osteolytic represents two extremes reflecting the altered functions of the osteoblasts, osteoclasts, and the coupling process between them [129,130].

Some malignancies such as breast and prostate cancers commonly metastasize to bone. Epidemiological data indicates that more than 80% of all men who die of prostate cancer have metastatic disease within bone and that about 75% of patients with advanced breast cancer develop bone metastases. Skeletal complications are also associated with multiple myeloma, a blood malignancy in which tumor cells lead to focal and diffuse osteolytic lesions. Bone metastasis also occurs in a significant number (15–40%) of patients with other types of solid tumors such as renal, thyroid, lung and colon cancers [131,132].

Prostate cancer has been described as an osteoblastic prototype tumor where prostate cancer cells produce numerous osteogenic factors resulting in primarily osteoblastic lesions. The mechanisms underlying this osteopenic component of prostate cancer–mediated bone lesions have not been fully elucidated. However, several proteins including endothelins and bone morphogenetic proteins have been hypothesized to play roles in the formation of osteoblastic lesions. Some growth factors produced by tumor cells such as platelet-derived growth factor, insulin-like growth factors, and adrenomedullin have also been implicated in osteoblastic bone metastases. [132]. Endothelin-1 (ET-1) is a vasoactive peptide that has been recently recognized as a stimulator for new bone formation associated with osteoblastic bone metastases via the endothelin A receptor (ETAR) in both mice and humans. Studies on patients with metastatic prostate cancer showed that ETAR antagonist reduced skeletal morbidity and has also been shown to prevent osteoblastic bone metastases in a mouse model [133-136].

Although prostate tumors are known to have expression of the osteolytic factor PTHrP, the mode of metastases to the skeleton is considered osteoblastic and a possible suggested explanation for this is that NH2-terminal fragments of PTHrP stimulate new bone formation by activating ETAR. The NH2-terminal peptides do not bind to ETAR when overexpressed in mammalian cells thus suggesting that an accessory receptor subunit is expressed in certain cell types such as osteoblasts making them responsive to these alternative ETAR ligands. Researchers propose that the mimicry of ET-1 by PTHrP NH2-terminal peptides means that ETAR antagonists could be effective in treating prostate cancer, both against the actions of endothelin itself and against the anabolic effects of PTHrP fragments [132].

Recent evidence has emerged that the altered regulation of RANKL and OPG is key to cancer related bone diseases. Studies in animal models bearing prostate tumors have shown that RANKL inhibition and subsequent osteoclast depletion slows the progression of osteoblastic lesions induced by prostate cancer cells. It also reduced bone turnover marker levels. The reduction in osteoblastic lesions after treatment with RANKL inhibitors correlated with a reduction in bone formation markers such as serum osteocalcin and bone specific alkaline phosphatase, as well as bone resorption marker such as the urine N-telopeptide of type I collagen (NTX) [130, 137-140]. OPG expression has also been reportedly altered in cancer cases. Increased serum OPG levels were correlated with the presence of bone metastases in breast and prostate cancer cases. Higher OPG levels were also linked to increased levels of bone resorption markers, which was suggested to be a compensatory response of osteoblasts to increased bone turnover. The data clearly demonstrated that osteoclast activity has been essential for the development of osteoblastic prostate tumors in bone. Therefore, it is proposed that blocking osteoclast activity and differentiation via RANKL inhibition may not only provide a beneficial treatment for skeletal complications of malignancy, but may also prevent bone metastases [141,142].

In conclusion, osteoblasts are responsible for the formation and maintenance of the skeletal architecture. They produce extracellular matrix proteins and regulate matrix mineralization during bone formation and remodeling. The need for a better understanding of the roles that osteoblasts and the signaling proteins that control them will lead to further advance our understanding of the mechanisms and pathogenesis of many skeletal disorders.

Acknowledgment

The authors would like to thank Elizabeth Smith for her help in the MG63 experiments.

References

[1] Siebers MC, ter Brugge PJ, Walboomers XF, Jansen JA: Integrins as linker proteins between osteoblasts and bone replacing materials. A critical review. *Biomaterials* 2005, 26(2):137-146.

[2] Steinemann SG: Titanium--the material of choice? *Periodontology* 2000 1998, 17:7-21.

[3] Ducy P, Schinke T, Karsenty G: The osteoblast: a sophisticated fibroblast under central surveillance. *Science* 2000, 289(5484):1501-1504.

[4] Seeman E, Delmas PD: Bone quality--the material and structural basis of bone strength and fragility. *The New England journal of medicine* 2006, 354(21):2250-2261.

[5] Noble B: Microdamage and apoptosis. *European journal of morphology* 2005, 42(1-2):91-98.

[6] Raisz LG, Kream BE: Regulation of bone formation. *The New England journal of medicine* 1983, 309(1):29-35.

[7] Gori F, Hofbauer LC, Dunstan CR, Spelsberg TC, Khosla S, Riggs BL: The expression of osteoprotegerin and RANK ligand and the support of osteoclast formation by stromal-osteoblast lineage cells is developmentally regulated. *Endocrinology* 2000, 141(12):4768-4776.

[8] Kristensen LP, Chen L, Nielsen MO, Qanie DW, Kratchmarova I, Kassem M, Andersen JS: Temporal profiling and pulsed SILAC labeling identify novel secreted proteins during ex vivo osteoblast differentiation of human stromal stem cells. *Molecular & cellular proteomics* : MCP 2012.

[9] Rached MT, Kode A, Silva BC, Jung DY, Gray S, Ong H, Paik JH, DePinho RA, Kim JK, Karsenty G et al: FoxO1 expression in osteoblasts regulates glucose homeostasis through regulation of osteocalcin in mice. *The Journal of clinical investigation* 2010, 120(1):357-368.

[10] Friedenstein AJ, Chailakhyan RK, Gerasimov UV: Bone marrow osteogenic stem cells: in vitro cultivation and transplantation in diffusion chambers. *Cell and tissue kinetics* 1987, 20(3):263-272.

[11] Yamaguchi A, Komori T, Suda T: Regulation of osteoblast differentiation mediated by bone morphogenetic proteins, hedgehogs, and Cbfa1. *Endocrine reviews* 2000, 21(4):393-411.

[12] Minguell JJ, Erices A, Conget P: Mesenchymal stem cells. Exp Biol Med (Maywood) 2001, 226(6):507-520.

[13] de Crombrugghe B, Lefebvre V, Behringer RR, Bi W, Murakami S, Huang W: Transcriptional mechanisms of chondrocyte differentiation. Matrix biology : journal of the International Society for Matrix Biology 2000, 19(5):389-394.

[14] Tontonoz P, Spiegelman BM: Fat and beyond: the diverse biology of PPARgamma. *Annual review of biochemistry* 2008, 77:289-312.

[15] Komori T, Yagi H, Nomura S, Yamaguchi A, Sasaki K, Deguchi K, Shimizu Y, Bronson RT, Gao YH, Inada M et al: Targeted disruption of Cbfa1 results in a complete lack of bone formation owing to maturational arrest of osteoblasts. *Cell* 1997, 89(5):755-764.

[16] Otto F, Thornell AP, Crompton T, Denzel A, Gilmour KC, Rosewell IR, Stamp GW, Beddington RS, Mundlos S, Olsen BR et al: Cbfa1, a candidate gene for cleidocranial dysplasia syndrome, is essential for osteoblast differentiation and bone development. *Cell* 1997, 89(5):765-771.

[17] Pittenger MF, Mackay AM, Beck SC, Jaiswal RK, Douglas R, Mosca JD, Moorman MA, Simonetti DW, Craig S, Marshak DR: Multilineage potential of adult human mesenchymal stem cells. *Science* 1999, 284(5411):143-147.

[18] Caplan AI: Mesenchymal stem cells. *Journal of orthopaedic research : official publication of the Orthopaedic Research Society* 1991, 9(5):641-650.

[19] Pelletier N, Champagne N, Stifani S, Yang XJ: MOZ and MORF histone acetyltransferases interact with the Runt-domain transcription factor Runx2. *Oncogene* 2002, 21(17):2729-2740.

[20] Stein GS, Lian JB, Gerstenfeld LG, Shalhoub V, Aronow M, Owen T, Markose E: The onset and progression of osteoblast differentiation is functionally related to cellular proliferation. *Connective tissue research* 1989, 20(1-4):3-13.

[21] Ambrosetti D, Holmes G, Mansukhani A, Basilico C: Fibroblast growth factor signaling uses multiple mechanisms to inhibit Wnt-induced transcription in osteoblasts. *Molecular and cellular biology* 2008, 28(15):4759-4771.

[22] Hu H, Hilton MJ, Tu X, Yu K, Ornitz DM, Long F: Sequential roles of Hedgehog and Wnt signaling in osteoblast development. *Development* 2005, 132(1):49-60.

[23] Mukherjee A, Rotwein P: Akt promotes BMP2-mediated osteoblast differentiation and bone development. *Journal of cell science* 2009, 122(Pt 5):716-726.

[24] Baumbach LL, Marashi F, Plumb M, Stein G, Stein J: Inhibition of DNA replication coordinately reduces cellular levels of core and H1 histone mRNAs: requirement for protein synthesis. *Biochemistry* 1984, 23(8):1618-1625.

[25] Buckley MJ, Banes AJ, Jordan RD: The effects of mechanical strain on osteoblasts in vitro. Journal of oral and maxillofacial surgery : official journal of the American Association of Oral and Maxillofacial Surgeons 1990, 48(3):276-282; discussion 282-273.

[26] Canalis E, Pash J, Varghese S: Skeletal growth factors. *Critical reviews in eukaryotic gene expression* 1993, 3(3):155-166.

[27] Cheng SL, Yang JW, Rifas L, Zhang SF, Avioli LV: Differentiation of human bone marrow osteogenic stromal cells in vitro: induction of the osteoblast phenotype by dexamethasone. *Endocrinology* 1994, 134(1):277-286.

[28] Nishio Y, Dong Y, Paris M, O'Keefe RJ, Schwarz EM, Drissi H: Runx2-mediated regulation of the zinc finger Osterix/Sp7 gene. *Gene* 2006, 372:62-70.

[29] Acampora D, Merlo GR, Paleari L, Zerega B, Postiglione MP, Mantero S, Bober E, Barbieri O, Simeone A, Levi G: Craniofacial, vestibular and bone defects in mice lacking the Distal-less-related gene Dlx5. *Development* 1999, 126(17):3795-3809.

[30] Bialek P, Kern B, Yang X, Schrock M, Sosic D, Hong N, Wu H, Yu K, Ornitz DM, Olson EN et al: A twist code determines the onset of osteoblast differentiation. *Developmental cell* 2004, 6(3):423-435.

[31] Dobreva G, Chahrour M, Dautzenberg M, Chirivella L, Kanzler B, Farinas I, Karsenty G, Grosschedl R: SATB2 is a multifunctional determinant of craniofacial patterning and osteoblast differentiation. *Cell* 2006, 125(5):971-986.

[32] Jones DC, Wein MN, Oukka M, Hofstaetter JG, Glimcher MJ, Glimcher LH: Regulation of adult bone mass by the zinc finger adapter protein Schnurri-3. *Science* 2006, 312(5777):1223-1227.

[33] Yang X, Matsuda K, Bialek P, Jacquot S, Masuoka HC, Schinke T, Li L, Brancorsini S, Sassone-Corsi P, Townes TM et al: ATF4 is a substrate of RSK2 and an essential regulator of osteoblast biology; implication for Coffin-Lowry Syndrome. *Cell* 2004, 117(3):387-398.

[34] Fujita T, Azuma Y, Fukuyama R, Hattori Y, Yoshida C, Koida M, Ogita K, Komori T: Runx2 induces osteoblast and chondrocyte differentiation and enhances their migration by coupling with PI3K-Akt signaling. *The Journal of cell biology* 2004, 166(1):85-95.

[35] Komori T: Regulation of skeletal development by the Runx family of transcription factors. *Journal of cellular biochemistry* 2005, 95(3):445-453.

[36] Kundu M, Chen A, Anderson S, Kirby M, Xu L, Castilla LH, Bodine D, Liu PP: Role of Cbfb in hematopoiesis and perturbations resulting from expression of the leukemogenic fusion gene Cbfb-MYH11. *Blood* 2002, 100(7):2449-2456.

[37] Tachibana M, Tenno M, Tezuka C, Sugiyama M, Yoshida H, Taniuchi I: Runx1/Cbfbeta2 complexes are required for lymphoid tissue inducer cell differentiation at two developmental stages. *J Immunol* 2011, 186(3):1450-1457.

[38] Lund AH, van Lohuizen M: RUNX: a trilogy of cancer genes. *Cancer cell* 2002, 1(3):213-215.

[39] Baniwal SK, Shah PK, Shi Y, Haduong JH, Declerck YA, Gabet Y, Frenkel B: Runx2 promotes both osteoblastogenesis and novel osteoclastogenic signals in ST2 mesenchymal progenitor cells. Osteoporosis international : a journal established as result of cooperation between the European Foundation for Osteoporosis and the National Osteoporosis Foundation of the USA 2012, 23(4):1399-1413.

[40] Shimoyama A, Wada M, Ikeda F, Hata K, Matsubara T, Nifuji A, Noda M, Amano K, Yamaguchi A, Nishimura R et al: Ihh/Gli2 signaling promotes osteoblast differentiation by regulating Runx2 expression and function. *Molecular biology of the cell* 2007, 18(7):2411-2418.

[41] Ducy P, Zhang R, Geoffroy V, Ridall AL, Karsenty G: Osf2/Cbfa1: a transcriptional activator of osteoblast differentiation. *Cell* 1997, 89(5):747-754.

[42] Martin JW, Zielenska M, Stein GS, van Wijnen AJ, Squire JA: The Role of RUNX2 in Osteosarcoma Oncogenesis. Sarcoma 2011, 2011:282745.

[43] van der Deen M, Akech J, Lapointe D, Gupta S, Young DW, Montecino MA, Galindo M, Lian JB, Stein JL, Stein GS et al: Genomic promoter occupancy of runt-related transcription factor RUNX2 in Osteosarcoma cells identifies genes involved in cell adhesion and motility. *The Journal of biological chemistry* 2012, 287(7):4503-4517.

[44] Lucero C, Vega O, Osorio M, Tapia JC, Antonelli M, Stein GS, van Wijnen AJ, Galindo M: The cancer-related transcription factor Runx2 modulates cell proliferation in human osteosarcoma cell lines. *Journal of cellular physiology* 2012.

[45] Nakashima K, Zhou X, Kunkel G, Zhang Z, Deng JM, Behringer RR, de Crombrugghe B: The novel zinc finger-containing transcription factor osterix is required for osteoblast differentiation and bone formation. *Cell* 2002, 108(1):17-29.

[46] Yang X, Karsenty G: ATF4, the osteoblast accumulation of which is determined post-translationally, can induce osteoblast-specific gene expression in non-osteoblastic cells. *The Journal of biological chemistry* 2004, 279(45):47109-47114.

[47] Xiao G, Jiang D, Ge C, Zhao Z, Lai Y, Boules H, Phimphilai M, Yang X, Karsenty G, Franceschi RT: Cooperative interactions between activating transcription factor 4 and Runx2/Cbfa1 stimulate osteoblast-specific osteocalcin gene expression. *The Journal of biological chemistry* 2005, 280(35):30689-30696.

[48] Yu S, Franceschi RT, Luo M, Zhang X, Jiang D, Lai Y, Jiang Y, Zhang J, Xiao G: Parathyroid hormone increases activating transcription factor 4 expression and activity in osteoblasts: requirement for osteocalcin gene expression. *Endocrinology* 2008, 149(4):1960-1968.

[49] Yu S, Franceschi RT, Luo M, Fan J, Jiang D, Cao H, Kwon TG, Lai Y, Zhang J, Patrene K et al: Critical role of activating transcription factor 4 in the anabolic actions of parathyroid hormone in bone. *PloS one* 2009, 4(10):e7583.

[50] Hariharan R, Pillai MR: Structure-function relationship of inhibitory Smads: Structural flexibility contributes to functional divergence. *Proteins* 2008, 71(4):1853-1862.

[51] Yang X, Chen L, Xu X, Li C, Huang C, Deng CX: TGF-beta/Smad3 signals repress chondrocyte hypertrophic differentiation and are required for maintaining articular cartilage. *The Journal of cell biology* 2001, 153(1):35-46.

[52] Tan X, Weng T, Zhang J, Wang J, Li W, Wan H, Lan Y, Cheng X, Hou N, Liu H et al: Smad4 is required for maintaining normal murine postnatal bone homeostasis. *Journal of cell science* 2007, 120(Pt 13):2162-2170.

[53] Meredith JE, Jr., Winitz S, Lewis JM, Hess S, Ren XD, Renshaw MW, Schwartz MA: The regulation of growth and intracellular signaling by integrins. *Endocrine reviews* 1996, 17(3):207-220.

[54] Schwartz MA, Schaller MD, Ginsberg MH: Integrins: emerging paradigms of signal transduction. *Annual review of cell and developmental biology* 1995, 11:549-599.

[55] Eleniste PP, Bruzzaniti A: Focal adhesion kinases in adhesion structures and disease. *Journal of signal transduction* 2012, 2012:296450.

[56] Clover J, Dodds RA, Gowen M: Integrin subunit expression by human osteoblasts and osteoclasts in situ and in culture. *Journal of cell science* 1992, 103 (Pt 1):267-271.

[57] Hughes DE, Salter DM, Dedhar S, Simpson R: Integrin expression in human bone. Journal of bone and mineral research : *the official journal of the American Society for Bone and Mineral Research* 1993, 8(5):527-533.

[58] Moursi AM, Globus RK, Damsky CH: Interactions between integrin receptors and fibronectin are required for calvarial osteoblast differentiation in vitro. *Journal of cell science* 1997, 110 (Pt 18):2187-2196.

[59] Gronthos S, Stewart K, Graves SE, Hay S, Simmons PJ: Integrin expression and function on human osteoblast-like cells. Journal of bone and mineral research : *the official journal of the American Society for Bone and Mineral Research* 1997, 12(8):1189-1197.

[60] Adams JC, Watt FM: Regulation of development and differentiation by the extracellular matrix. *Development* 1993, 117(4):1183-1198.

[61] Liu YK, Uemura T, Nemoto A, Yabe T, Fujii N, Ushida T, Tateishi T: Osteopontin involvement in integrin-mediated cell signaling and regulation of expression of alkaline phosphatase during early differentiation of UMR cells. *FEBS letters* 1997, 420(1):112-116.

[62] Xiao G, Wang D, Benson MD, Karsenty G, Franceschi RT: Role of the alpha2-integrin in osteoblast-specific gene expression and activation of the Osf2 transcription factor. *The Journal of biological chemistry* 1998, 273(49):32988-32994.

[63] Lynch MP, Stein JL, Stein GS, Lian JB: The influence of type I collagen on the development and maintenance of the osteoblast phenotype in primary and passaged rat calvarial osteoblasts: modification of expression of genes supporting cell growth, adhesion, and extracellular matrix mineralization. *Experimental cell research* 1995, 216(1):35-45.

[64] Koch FP, Wunsch A, Merkel C, Ziebart T, Pabst A, Yekta SS, Blessmann M, Smeets R: The influence of bisphosphonates on human osteoblast migration and integrin aVb3/tenascin C gene expression in vitro. *Head & face medicine* 2011, 7(1):4.
[65] Hinshaw JE: Dynamin and its role in membrane fission. *Annual review of cell and developmental biology* 2000, 16:483-519.
[66] Song BD, Schmid SL: A molecular motor or a regulator? Dynamin's in a class of its own. *Biochemistry* 2003, 42(6):1369-1376.
[67] Schmid SL, McNiven MA, De Camilli P: Dynamin and its partners: a progress report. *Current opinion in cell biology* 1998, 10(4):504-512.
[68] Oh P, McIntosh DP, Schnitzer JE: Dynamin at the neck of caveolae mediates their budding to form transport vesicles by GTP-driven fission from the plasma membrane of endothelium. *The Journal of cell biology* 1998, 141(1):101-114.
[69] Werbonat Y, Kleutges N, Jakobs KH, van Koppen CJ: Essential role of dynamin in internalization of M2 muscarinic acetylcholine and angiotensin AT1A receptors. *J Biol Chem* 2000, 275(29):21969-21974.
[70] Kolokoltsov AA, Deniger D, Fleming EH, Roberts NJ, Jr., Karpilow JM, Davey RA: Small interfering RNA profiling reveals key role of clathrin-mediated endocytosis and early endosome formation for infection by respiratory syncytial virus. *Journal of virology* 2007, 81(14):7786-7800.
[71] Ochoa GC, Slepnev VI, Neff L, Ringstad N, Takei K, Daniell L, Kim W, Cao H, McNiven M, Baron R et al: A functional link between dynamin and the actin cytoskeleton at podosomes. *The Journal of cell biology* 2000, 150(2):377-389.
[72] Bruzzaniti A, Neff L, Sanjay A, Horne WC, De Camilli P, Baron R: Dynamin forms a Src kinase-sensitive complex with Cbl and regulates podosomes and osteoclast activity. *Molecular biology of the cell* 2005, 16(7):3301-3313.
[73] Eleniste PP, Du L, Shivanna M, Bruzzaniti A: Dynamin and PTP-PEST cooperatively regulate Pyk2 dephosphorylation in osteoclasts. *The international journal of biochemistry & cell biology* 2012, 44(5):790-800.
[74] Zamir E, Geiger B: Components of cell-matrix adhesions. *Journal of cell science* 2001, 114(Pt 20):3577-3579.
[75] Raisz LA. Pathogeneis of osteoporosis: concepts, conflicts, and prospects. *J Clin Invest* 2005, 115:3318–3325
[76] Beil FT, Seitz S, Priemel M, Barvencik F, Von Domuras C, Rueger JM, Amling M, Podoga P. Pathophysiology and pathomorphology of osteoporosis. *Eur J Trauma Emerg Surg* 2008, 6:527–534
[77] Neve A, Corrado A, Cantatore FP. Osteoblast physiology in normal and pathological conditions. *Cell Tissue Res* 2011, 343:289–302
[78] Phan TCA, Xu J, Zheng MH. Interaction between osteoblast and osteoclast: impact in bone disease. *Histol Histopathol* 2004, 19: 1325-1344
[79] Harada S, Rodan G. Control of osteoblast function and regulation of bone mass. *Nature* 2003, 423:349-355
[80] Benson BW, Shulman JD. Inclusion of tobacco exposure as a predictive factor for decreased bone mineral content. *Nicotine Tob Res* 2005, 7:719–724
[81] Kapoor D, Jones TH. Smoking and hormones in health and endocrine disorders. *Eur J Endocrinol* 2005, 152:491–499

[82] Giuliani N, Girasole G, Vescovi PP, Passeri G, Pedrazzoni M. Ethanol and acetaldehyde inhibit the formation of early osteoblast progenitors in murine and human bone marrow cultures. *Alcohol Clin Exp Res* 1999, 23:381–385

[83] Rodríguez JP, Astudillo P, Ríos S, Pino AM. Involvement of adipogenic potential of human bone marrow mesenchymal stem cells (MSCs) in osteoporosis. *Curr Stem Cell Res Ther* 2008, 3:208–218

[84] Perrini S, Natalicchio A, Laviola L, Cignarelli A, Melchiorre M, De Stefano F, Caccioppoli C, Leonardini A, Martemucci S,Belsanti G, Miccoli S, Ciampolillo A, Corrado A, Cantatore FP, Giorgino R, Giorgino F. Abnormalities of insulin-like growth factor-I signaling and impaired cell proliferation in osteoblasts from subjects with osteoporosis. *Endocrinology* 2008, 149:1302–1313

[85] Maruotti N, Corrado A, Grano M, Colucci S, Cantatore FP.Normal and osteoporotic human osteoblast behaviour after 1, 25- dihydroxy-vitamin D(3) stimulation. *Rheumatol Int* 2009, 29:667–672

[86] Torricelli P, Fini M, Giavaresi G, Giardino R. Human osteoblast cultures from osteoporotic and healthy bone: biochemical markers and cytokine expression in basal conditions and in response to 1, 25(OH)2D3. *Artif Cells Blood Substit Immobil Biotechnol* 2002, 30:219–227

[87] Neidlinger-Wilke C, Stalla I, Claes L, Brand R, Hoellen I, Rübenacker S, Arand M, Kinzl L. Human osteoblasts from younger normal and osteoporotic donors show differences in proliferation and TGF beta-release in response to cyclic strain. *J Biomech* 1995, 28:1411–1418

[88] Troen BR. Molecular mechanisms underlying osteoclast formation and activation. *Exp. Gerontol* 2003, 38: 605-614.

[89] Hofbauer LC, Khosla S, Dunstan CR, Lacey DL, Spelsberg TC, Riggs BL. Estrogen stimulates gene expression and protein production of osteoprotegerin in human osteoblastic cells. *Endocrinology* 1999,140: 4367-4370.

[90] Khosla S, Atkinson EJ, Dunstan CR, O'Fallon WM. Effect of estrogen versus testosterone on circulating osteoprotegerin and other cytokine levels in normal elderly men. *J Clin Endocrinol Metab* 2002, 87: 1550-1544.

[91] Shevde NK, Bendixen AC, Dienger KM, Pike JW. Estrogens suppress rank ligand-induced osteoclast differentiation via a stromal cell independent mechanism involving c-jun repression. *Proc Natl Acad Sci* 2000, 97: 7829-7834.

[92] Krishnan V, Bryant HU, Macdougald OA. Regulation of bone mass by Wnt signaling. *J Clin Invest* 2006, 116: 1202–1209.

[93] Johnson ML, Harnish K, Nusse R, Van Hul W. LRP5 and Wnt signaling: a union made for bone. *J Bone Min Res* 2004, 19: 1749–1757.

[94] Bodine PV, Komm BS. Wnt signaling and osteoblastogenesis. *Reviews in Endocrine and Metabolic Disorders* 2006, 7: 33–39.

[95] Rawadi G, Vayssiere B, Dunn F, Baron R, Roman-Roman S. BMP-2 controls alkaline phosphatase expression and osteoblast mineralization by a Wnt autocrine loop. *J Bone Min Res* 2003, 18: 1842–1853.

[96] Kramer I, Keller H, Leupin O, Kneissel M. Does osteocytic SOST suppression mediate PTH bone anabolism? *Trends in Endocrin Metabol* 2010, 21: 237–244.

[97] Manolagas SC, Almeida M. Gone with the Wnts: beta-catenin, T-cell factor, forkhead box O, and oxidative stress in age-dependent diseases of bone, lipid, and glucose metabolism. *Mol Endocrinol* 2007, 21: 2605–2614.

[98] Robinson JA, Chatterjee-Kishore M, Yaworsky PJ, Cullen DM, Zhao W, Li C, Kharode Y, Sauter L, Babij P, Brown EL, Hill AA, Akhter MP, Johnson ML, Recker RR, Komm BS, Bex FJ. Wnt/beta-catenin signaling is a normal physiological response to mechanical loading in bone. *J Biol Chem* 2006, 281: 31720–31728.

[99] Clement-Lacroix P, Ai M, Morvan F, Roman-Roman S, Vayssiere B, Belleville C, Estrera K, Warman ML, Baron R, Rawadi G. Lrp5-independent activation of Wnt signaling by lithium chloride increases bone formation and bone mass in mice. *PNAS* 2005, 102: 17406–17411.

[100] Kulkarni NH, Onyia JE, Zeng Q, Tian X, Liu M, Halladay DL, Frolik CA, Engler T, Wei T, Kriauciunas A, Martin TJ, Sato M, Bryant HU & Ma YL. Orally bioavailable GSK-3alpha/beta dual inhibitor increases markers of cellular differentiation in vitro and bone mass in vivo. *J Bone Miner Res* 2006, 21: 910–920.

[101] Li X, Ominsky MS, Warmington KS, Morony S, Gong J, Cao J, Gao Y, Shalhoub V, Tipton B, Haldankar R, Chen Q, Winters A, Boone T, Geng Z, Niu QT, Ke HZ, Kostenuik PJ, Simonet WS, Lacey DL, Paszty C. Sclerostin antibody treatment increases bone formation, bone mass, and bone strength in a rat model of postmenopausal osteoporosis. *J Bone Miner Res* 2009, 24: 578–588.

[102] Padhi D, Jang G, Stouch B, Fang L, Posvar E. Single-dose, placebo-controlled, randomized study of AMG 785, a sclerostin monoclonal antibody. *J Bone Miner Res* 2011, 26: 19–26.

[103] Morvan F, Boulukos K, Clement-Lacroix P, Roman Roman S, Suc-Royer I, Vayssiere B, Ammann P, Martin P, Pinho S, Pognonec P, Mollat P, Niehrs C, Baron R, Rawadi G. Deletion of a single allele of the Dkk1 gene leads to an increase in bone formation and bone mass. *J Bone Miner Res* 2006, 21: 934–945.

[104] Guo J, Liu M, Yang D, Bouxsein ML, Saito H, Galvin RJ, Kuhstoss SA, Thomas CC, Schipani E, Baron R, Bringhurst FR, Kronenberg HM. Suppression of Wnt signaling by Dkk1 attenuates PTH-mediated stromal cell response and new bone formation. *Cell Metabolism* 2010, 11: 161–171.

[105] Yao W, Cheng Z, Shahnazari M, Dai W, Johnson ML, Lane NE. Overexpression of secreted frizzled-related protein 1 inhibits bone formation and attenuates PTH bone anabolic effects. *J Bone Miner Res* 2010, 25: 190–199.

[106] Bucay N, Sarosi I, Dunstan CR, Morony S, Tarpley J, Capparelli C, Scully S, Tan HL, Xu W, Lacey DL, Boyle WJ, Simonet WS. Osteoprotegerin-deficient mice develop early onset osteoporosis and arterial calcification. *Genes Dev* 1998, 12:1260–1268

[107] Eghbali-Fatourechi G, Khosla S, Sanyal A, Boyle WJ, Lacey DL, Riggs B. Role of RANK ligand in mediating increased bone resorption in early postmenopausal women. *J Clin Invest* 2003, 111:1221–1230

[108] Bekker PJ, Holloway DL, Rasmussen AS, Murphy R, Martin SW, Leese PT, Holmes GB, Dunstan CR, DePaoli AM. A single-dose placebo-controlled study of AMG 162, a fully human monoclonal antibody to RANKL, in postmenopausal women. *J Bone Miner Res* 2004, 19:1059–1066

[109] El Miedany YM, Mehanna AN, El Baddini MA. Altered bone mineral metabolism in patients with osteoarthritis. *Joint Bone Spine* 2000, 67:521–527

[110] Hilal G, Martel-Pelletier J, Pelletier JP, Ranger P, Lajeunesse D. Osteoblast-like cells from human subchondral osteoarthritic bone demonstrate an altered phenotype in vitro: possible role in subchondral bone sclerosis. *Arthritis Rheum* 1998, 41:891–899

[111] Lajeunesse D, Reboul P. Subchondral bone in osteoarthritis: a biologic link with articular cartilage leading to abnormal remodeling. *Curr Opin Rheumatol* 2003, 15:628–633

[112] Mansell JP, Bailey AJ. Abnormal cancellous bone collagen metabolism in osteoarthritis. *J Clin Invest* 1998, 101:1596–1603

[113] Couchourel D, Aubry I, Delalandre A, Lavigne M, Martel-Pelletier J, Pelletier JP, Lajeunesse D. Altered mineralization of human osteoarthritic osteoblasts is attributable to abnormal type I collagen production. *Arthritis Rheum* 2009, 60:1438–1450

[114] Kwan Tat S, Pelletier JP, Amiable N, Boileau C, Lajeunesse D, Duval N, Martel-Pelletier J. Activation of the receptor EphB4 by its specific ligand ephrin B2 in human osteoarthritic subchondral bone osteoblasts. *Arthritis Rheum* 2008, 58:3820–3830

[115] Glorieux F. A disease of the osteoblast. *The Lancet Suppl* 2001, 358: s45.

[116] Owen RH. Van Buchem's disease. *Br J Radiol* 1976, 49:126-132

[117] Hul WV, Balemans W, Hul EV, Dikkers FG, Obee H, Stokroos R, Hildering P, Vanhoenacker F, Camp GV, Willems P. Van Buchem diseade (Hyperstosis Corticalis Generalisata) maps to chromosome 17q12-q21. *Am J Hum Genet* 1998, 62: 391-399

[118] Brunkow ME, Gardner JC, Van Ness J, Paeper BW, Kovacevich BR, Proll S, Skonier JE, Zhao L, Sabo PJ, Fu Y et al: Bone dysplasia sclerosteosis results from loss of the SOST gene product, a novel cystine knot-containing protein. *Am J Hum Genet* 2001, 68(3):577-589.

[119] Sutherland MK, Geoghegan JC, Yu C, Winkler DG, Latham JA: Unique regulation of SOST, the sclerosteosis gene, by BMPs and steroid hormones in human osteoblasts. *Bone* 2004, 35(2):448-454.

[120] McLachlan E, Plante I, Shao Q, Tong D, Kidder GM, Bernier SM, Laird DW: ODDD-linked Cx43 mutants reduce endogenous Cx43 expression and function in osteoblasts and inhibit late stage differentiation. *J Bone Miner Res* 2008, 23:928-938.

[121] Pernow Y, Granberg B, Saaf M, Weidenhielm L: Osteoblast dysfunction in male idiopathic osteoporosis. *Calcified tissue international* 2006, 78:90-97.

[122] Sezer O: Myeloma bone disease: recent advances in biology, diagnosis, and treatment. *The oncologist* 2009, 14(3):276-283.

[123] Furlan F, Lecanda F, Screen J, Civitelli R: Proliferation, differentiation and apoptosis in connexin43-null osteoblasts. *Cell communication & adhesion* 2001, 8:367-371.

[124] Lecanda F, Warlow PM, Sheikh S, Furlan F, Steinberg TH, Civitelli R: Connexin43 deficiency causes delayed ossification, craniofacial abnormalities, and osteoblast dysfunction. *J Cell Biol* 151:931-944.

[125] Chung DJ, Castro CH, Watkins M, Stains JP, Chung MY, Szejnfeld VL, Willecke K, Theis M, Civitelli R: Low peak bone mass and attenuated anabolic response to parathyroid hormone in mice with an osteoblast-specific deletion of connexin43. *J CellSci* 2006, 119:4187-4198.

[126] Loiselle AE, Paul EM, Lewis GS, Donahue HJ: Osteoblast and osteocyte-specific loss of Connexin43 results in delayed bone formation and healing during murine fracture healing. *J Orthop Res* 2012, doi: 10.1002/jor.22178.

[127] Wu S, Liang S, Yan Y, Wang Y, Li F, Deng Y, Huang W, Yuan W, Luo N, Zhu C et al: A novel mutation of TGF beta1 in a Chinese family with Camurati-Engelmann disease. *Bone* 2007, 40:1630-1634.

[128] Romer P, Behr M, Proff P, Faltermeier A, Reicheneder C: Effect of strontium on human Runx2+/- osteoblasts from a patient with cleidocranial dysplasia. *Eur J Phama* 2011, 654:195-199.

[129] Coleman RE. Skeletal complications of malignancy. *Cancer* 2006, 80: 1588–1594

[130] Dougall WC, Chaisson M. The RANK/RANKL/OPG triad in cancer-induced bone diseases. *Cancer Metastasis Rev* (2006) 25:541–549

[131] Roodman GD. Mechanisms of bone metastasis. *New England Journal of Medicine* 2004, 350: 1655–1664.

[132] Guise TA,Mohammad KS,Clines G, Stebbins EG, Wong DH, Higgins LS,Vessella R, Corey E, Padalecki S, Suva L, Chirgwin J. Basic mechanisms responsible for osteolytic and osteoblastic bone metastases. *Clin Cancer Res* 2006, 12: 6213-6216.

[133] Nelson J, BagnatoA, Battistini B, Nisen P.The endothelin axis: emerging role in cancer. *Nat Rev Cancer* 2003,3:110-16.

[134] Yin JJ, Mohammad KS, Kakonen SM, et al. A causal role for endothelin-1in the pathogenesis of osteoblastic bone metastases. *Proc Natl Acad* Sci 2003, 100:10954-9.

[135] Nelson JB, Hedican SP, George DJ. Identification of endothelin-1 in the pathophysiology of metastatic adenocarcinoma of the prostate. *Nat Med* 1995;1:944-9.

[136] Carducci MA, Padley RJ, Breul J. Effect of endothelin-A receptor blockade with atrasentan on tumor progression in men with hormone-refractory prostate cancer: a randomized, phase II, placebocontrolled trial. *JClin Oncol* 2003,21:679-89.

[137] Brown JM, Corey E, Lee ZD, True LD, Yun TJ, Tondravi M. Osteoprotegerin and rank ligand expression in prostate cancer. *Urology* 2001, 57: 611–616.

[138] Granchi D, Amato I, Battistelli L, Avnet S, Capaccioli S, Papucci L. In vitro blockade of receptor activator of nuclear factor-kappaB ligand prevents osteoclastogenesis induced by neuroblastoma cells. *Int J Canc* 2004, 111: 829–838.

[139] Farrugia AN, Atkins GJ, To LB, Pan B, Horvath N, Kostakis P. Receptor activator of nuclear factorkappaB ligand expression by human myeloma cells mediates osteoclast formation in vitro and correlates with bone destruction in vivo. *Cancer Res* 2003, 63: 5438–5445.

[140] Blair JM, Zhou H, Seibel MJ, Dunstan CR. Mechanisms of disease: Roles of OPG, RANKL and RANK in the pathophysiology of skeletal metastasis. *Nat Clin Pract Oncol* 2006, 3: 41–49.

[141] Dovio A, Data V, Angeli A. Circulating osteoprotegerin and soluble RANKL: Do they have a future in clinical practice? *J Endocrinol Invest* 2005, 28(Suppl 10): 14–22.

[142] Holen I, Croucher PI, Hamdy FC, Eaton CL. Osteoprotegerin (OPG) is a survival factor for human prostate cancer cells. *Cancer Res* 2002, 62: 1619–1623.

[143] Day TF, Guo X, Garrett-Beal L, Yang Y: Wnt/beta-catenin signaling in mesenchymal progenitors controls osteoblast and chondrocyte differentiation during vertebrate skeletogenesis. *Developmental cell* 2005, 8(5):739-750.

[144] Hill TP, Spater D, Taketo MM, Birchmeier W, Hartmann C: Canonical Wnt/beta-catenin signaling prevents osteoblasts from differentiating into chondrocytes. *Developmental cell* 2005, 8(5):727-738.

[145] Rodda SJ, McMahon AP: Distinct roles for Hedgehog and canonical Wnt signaling in specification, differentiation and maintenance of osteoblast progenitors. *Development* 2006, 133(16):3231-3244.
[146] Glass DA, 2nd, Bialek P, Ahn JD, Starbuck M, Patel MS, Clevers H, Taketo MM, Long F, McMahon AP, Lang RA et al: Canonical Wnt signaling in differentiated osteoblasts controls osteoclast differentiation. *Developmental cell* 2005, 8(5):751-764.
[147] Koga T, Matsui Y, Asagiri M, Kodama T, de Crombrugghe B, Nakashima K, Takayanagi H: NFAT and Osterix cooperatively regulate bone formation. *Nature medicine* 2005, 11(8):880-885.
[148] Zhang C: Transcriptional regulation of bone formation by the osteoblast-specific transcription factor Osx. *Journal of orthopaedic surgery and research* 2010, 5:37.
[149] Wang W, Lian N, Ma Y, Li L, Gallant RC, Elefteriou F, Yang X: Chondrocytic Atf4 regulates osteoblast differentiation and function via Ihh. Development 2011.
[150] Iwai T, Murai J, Yoshikawa H, Tsumaki N: Smad7 Inhibits chondrocyte differentiation at multiple steps during endochondral bone formation and down-regulates p38 MAPK pathways. *The Journal of biological chemistry* 2008, 283(40):27154-27164.
[151] Zhang J, Tan X, Li W, Wang Y, Wang J, Cheng X, Yang X: Smad4 is required for the normal organization of the cartilage growth plate. *Developmental biology* 2005, 284(2):311-322.
[152] Wang M, Jin H, Tang D, Huang S, Zuscik MJ, Chen D: Smad1 plays an essential role in bone development and postnatal bone formation. Osteoarthritis and cartilage / OARS, Osteoarthritis Research Society 2011, 19(6):751-762.
[153] Lee MH, Kwon TG, Park HS, Wozney JM, Ryoo HM: BMP-2-induced Osterix expression is mediated by Dlx5 but is independent of Runx2. *Biochemical and biophysical research communications* 2003, 309(3):689-694.
[154] Robledo RF, Rajan L, Li X, Lufkin T: The Dlx5 and Dlx6 homeobox genes are essential for craniofacial, axial, and appendicular skeletal development. *Genes & development* 2002, 16(9):1089-1101.
[155] Kim YJ, Lee MH, Wozney JM, Cho JY, Ryoo HM: Bone morphogenetic protein-2-induced alkaline phosphatase expression is stimulated by Dlx5 and repressed by Msx2. *The Journal of biological chemistry* 2004, 279(49):50773-50780.
[156] Shu B, Zhang M, Xie R, Wang M, Jin H, Hou W, Tang D, Harris SE, Mishina Y, O'Keefe RJ et al: BMP2, but not BMP4, is crucial for chondrocyte proliferation and maturation during endochondral bone development. *Journal of cell science* 2011, 124(Pt 20):3428-3440.
[157] Bandyopadhyay A, Tsuji K, Cox K, Harfe BD, Rosen V, Tabin CJ: Genetic analysis of the roles of BMP2, BMP4, and BMP7 in limb patterning and skeletogenesis. *PLoS genetics* 2006, 2(12):e216.
[158] Alliston T, Choy L, Ducy P, Karsenty G, Derynck R: TGF-beta-induced repression of CBFA1 by Smad3 decreases cbfa1 and osteocalcin expression and inhibits osteoblast differentiation. *The EMBO journa*l 2001, 20(9):2254-2272.

In: Osteoblasts
Editor: Hugo Scheurer

ISBN: 978-1-62417-806-1

Chapter 4

Osteoblast Differentiation and Related Diseases

Juliana Marulanda*
Faculty of Dentistry, McGill University, Montreal, Quebec, Canada

Abstract

Bone-forming osteoblasts differentiate from the pluripotent mesenchymal stem cells (MSCs), through a cascade of signalling events that involves modulation of gene expression regulated by several key transcription factors. The first transcription factor and the master regulator of osteoblast differentiation is the Runt-related transcription factor 2 or RUNX2. Its expression in common chondro/osteoprogenitors is controlled by different homeodomain transcription factors and suppressors. RUNX2 not only plays a critical role in the early stages of development, but regulates bone formation beyond this phase. In differentiating osteoblasts, RUNX2 induces the expression of Osterix (OSX/SP7) an osteoblast-specific transcription factor. In genetic experiments, *Osx* inactivation in mice results in perinatal lethality, undifferentiated osteoblasts and complete absence of endochondral and intramembranous bone formation. Once committed, preosteoblasts become functional mainly because of ATF4 transcriptional activity which regulates the synthesis and secretion of type I collagen.

Genetic mutations leading to impaired osteoblastogenesis have been associated with several human diseases. A heterozygous mutation of the human *RUNX2* gene causes Cleidocranial dysplasia (CCD), condition characterized by a delay in fontanelles closure and hypoplasic clavicles. Recently, a single base pair mutation in the *SP7/OSX* gene was associated to a form of non-collagenous osteogenesis imperfecta characterized mainly by facial dysmorphism and frequent bone fractures, whereas a loss-of-function mutation in the *RSK2* gene leads to Coffin-Lowry syndrome, an X-linked condition that displays mental retardation and skeletal abnormalities in the affected males.

---

* Corresponding author: Juliana Marulanda, Address: 1529 Cedar Avenue Montreal, Quebec H3G 1A4, Canada E-mail: juliana.marulanda@mail.mcgill.ca, Phone: (514) 282-7167, Fax: (514) 842-5581.

This review will discuss the key transcription factors involved in osteoblast differentiation and the molecular mechanism of the genetic diseases caused by mutations in these regulatory genes.

Introduction

The synthesis and deposition of bone matrix and its subsequent mineralization is actively regulated by osteoblasts, the bone forming cells. Osteoblast progenitors differentiate from the pluripotent mesenchymal stem cells.

Although these progenitor cells in the craniofacial, axial and limb skeletons originate from different embryonic lineages —the neural crest, paraxial and lateral plate mesoderm, respectively, their terminal differentiation involves the same signaling events and downstream transcription factors.

Our current understanding of the regulation of the molecular events that regulate osteoblastogenesis is largely based on findings obtained from gene targeted mouse models and that from patients with congenital skeletal defects. Over the past twenty years, the advances in gene manipulation techniques have made mouse a very attractive model organism to study skeletal biology as the phenotypic consequences of gene mutations that affect skeletal development and functions are largely the same in mouse and human.

The current review will primarily focus on the *in vitro* and *in vivo* experimental data to provide a brief account of the major transcription factors that are invoved in osteoblast differentiation and also discuss about relevant human diseases that are associated with the muations in the genes encoding these transcription factors.

A. Transcription Factors Regulating Osteoblast Differentiation

RUNX2

It is imperative that the search for an osteoblast-specific transcription factor involves the analysis of a promoter that is active primarily in osteoblasts. The analysis of the regulatory elements in osteocalcin (*Bglap1*) promoter was therefore a logical step for this purpose. Indeed, classical promoter analysis experiments revealed a cis-acting element in the osteocalcin promoter and identified a nuclear protein that binds to it. This cis-acting element was named as Osteoblast-Specific Element 2 (OSE2) and the nuclear protein was initially named as Osteoblast-Specific Factor 2 (OSF2). Subsequent immunological studies showed that this factor is related to the transcription factors belonging to the Core Binding Factor (CBF) family [1]. CBF transcription factors are homologous to Drosophila Runts that were shown to play roles in neurogenesis, sexual differentiation and patterning during embryonic development [2]. In mammals, three runt homologues have been identified, which share a conserved 128 amino-acid RUNT DNA-binding domain, but show distinct functional roles in the regulation of neurogenesis, eye development, hematopoiesis and skeletal development [3].

OSF2/CBFA1 or RUNX2 was found to be a major transcriptional regulator for both osteoblast differentiation [4] and chondrocyte maturation [5].

In mice, three RUNX2 isoforms Type I, II and III have been identified. These isoforms carry distinct N-terminal sequences and have different transactivation potentials. The isoform Type I appears to be present in both osseous and non-osseous tissues including in liver, lung, muscle and skin; whereas the Type II and III are found primarily in terminal hypertrophic chondrocytes and in differentiated osteoblasts [6-8]. Interestingly, although the mRNAs encoding different RUNX2 isoforms are detected in multiple non-osteoblastic cells, osteoblast precursors and matured osteoblasts, no RUNX2 protein is detected in the former two cell types. This observation suggests that *Runx2* gene expression is regulated at the translational level [6].

During mouse development, *Runx2* expression reaches its pick in the chondro/osteo progenitor cells present in the condensed skeletal mesenchyme of 12.5 days post coitum (dpc) embryos. Thereafter, the first ossification center is formed at 14.5 dpc and *Runx2* expression is mostly detected in the differentiated osteoblasts. By 16 dpc only weaker *Runx2* expression is detected in prehypertrophic and hypertrophic chondrocytes but not in proliferating chondrocytes [1,9].

In order to understand the role of RUNX2 in osteoblast differentiation and bone formation, the *Runx2* knockout mice was generated by two independent groups in 1997. In both instances, the knockout mice died within few minutes after the birth due to respiratory failure. Their body weight represented 80% of the WT mice and staining of the skeleton with Alizarin red and X-Ray analysis indicated a weak calcification in tibia, radius and vertebra, whereas other bones did not show mineralization at all. To assess osteoblast maturation, the expression of Ostepontin, Oscteocalcin, Osteonectin and ALPL was determined. Osteonectin and ALPL were expressed in a low level whereas Osteopontin and Osteocalcin were almost undetected, which confirms that the arrest of osteoblast differentiation occurs at an early stage in RUNX2-deficient mice. *Runx2+/-* embryos and newborn mice exhibited a normal mineralization except for the absence of clavicles and impaired mineralization in cranium with open anterior and posterior fontanelle, phenotype that models the Cleidocranial dysplasia disease in humans [10,11].

Although the initial stages of cartilage formation appeared to be normal, the terminal differentiation of the chondrocytes was affected in *Runx2* knockout mice [11]. Analysis by *in-situ* hybridization revealed a lack of hypertrophic chondrocytes in the anlagen of humerus and phalanges and a delayed chondrocyte hypertrophy in radius and ulna of the null embryos [5]. Interestingly, the late chondrogenic markers such as Type X collagen, BMP6 and Indian hedgehog were expressed in the hypertrophic chondrocytes of the null embryos, although, Osteopontin, Bone sialoprotein and Collagenase III showed no expression. These results indicated that RUNX2 is required for the terminal differentiation of hypertrophic chondrocytes [12,13]. To further study the role of RUNX2 in late stage chondrocytes, *Col2a1* promoter driven continuous *Runx2* expression was induced in proliferating and prehypertrophic chondrocytes. There was an early chondrocyte hypertrophy and ectopic endochondral ossification in the cartilaginous tissues of these transgenic mice [14]. In agreement with these findings, selective ablation of *Runx2* in chondrocytes in mice, led to a disruption in chondrocyte differentiation and periosteal bone formation, resulting in shorter limbs [15, 16].

The role of RUNX2 in postnatal bone formation was evaluated in a transgenic model that overexpressed a RUNX2 DNA binding domain lacking the transactivation activity. As shown by Ducy *et al*, osteocalcin promoter driven expression of this dominant negative form of RUNX2 resulted in mice with normal skeletons at birth. However, after two weeks of age shorter stature of the transgenic mice became apparent and further analysis revealed osteopenic bones caused by a significant reduction in bone formation rate. Interestingly, unlike *Runx2-/-* mice, osteoblast numbers were normal in the dominant negative RUNX2 overexpressors [17]. Later, bone marrow ablation studies performed at 2.5 and 7.5 month-old *Runx2+/-* mice showed a reduction in bone formation especially in the aged mice. This result further establishes that full gene dosage of RUNX2 is required for normal bone formation in adult mice [18]. Based on these findings it was surprizing to note that overexpression of the full-length *Runx2* in the osteoblasts of the transgenic mice caused progressive decrease of bone mass. This apparently contradictory finding was explained by an increase of bone resorption as a result of increased expression of Collagenase 3 and Receptor Activator of NF-KappaB ligand (RANKL), two factors involved in osteoclastogenesis and bone resorption [19].

TWIST1

As described above, although *Runx2* expression in the condensed skeletal mesenchyme reaches its pick at 12.5 dpc, the first ossification center does not appear until 14.5 dpc. This suggests that there is an inhibition of RUNX2 function prior to the appearance of the well-defined skeletal tissues. Indeed, identification of a novel *Runx2*-interacting transcription factor TWIST1 and its functional analysis validated this insight. *Twist1* encodes a protein that contains a basic helix-loop-helix (b-HLH) motif, which was first identified in Drosophila, where it is responsible for the establishment of the germ layers [20]. In vertebrates, there are two of *Twist* homologues, *Twist1* and *Twist2*. Both TWIST1 and 2 carry a conserved C-terminus domain called the "Twist box" that binds to an E-box DNA motif found in promoters that regulate cell-specific gene transcription. TWIST1 has been shown to regulate neural tube and craniofacial development in mice and humans.

In mice, *Twist1* is first expressed at embryonic day 7.5 in the anterior-lateral mesoderm underlying the head folds. Later during embryonic development it is highly expressed in the mesenchymal cells of the head and branchial arches, but not in the ectoderm. After birth, *Twist1* expression has been detected in the pre-osteoblastic cells of calvaria which suggests its role in craniofacial mesenchymal development. Indeed, in agreement with TWIST1 expression pattern, analysis of the *Twist1*-null embryos shows incomplete closure of the neural crest, defects in head mesenchyme, branchial arches, somites and limb buds, although the posterior hindbrain and spinal cord appear to be normal. These findings suggest that TWIST1 is essential for head mesenchyme development. [21].

Twist1 has been identified as a major regulator in osteoblast differentiation. The overexpression of human *TWIST1* in SaOS-2 cells (human osteoblast-like sarcoma cells) resulted in a change of phenotype between the expressing cells and the control. Forced *TWIST1* expression in these cells kept them in an undifferentiated state and changed their morphology from a cuboidal-osteoblast shape to a spindle fibroblast phenotype. Additionally, there was a reduced expression of osteoblast markers such as Alkaline phosphatase and Type

I collagen and a decreased cell proliferation, further suggesting TWIST as a negative regulator of bone cell differentiation [22, 23]. Later on, in vivo studies showed that *Twist1* expression gradually decreases in developing mouse embryos prior to bone formation and concomitantly there is an induction of bone sialoprotein expression in the differentiating osteoblasts. Molecular biology experiments convincingly established a physical interaction between RUNX2 and TWIST1 and a functional inhibition of RUNX2-mediated gene expression by TWIST1. Finally, loss of one allele of TWIST1 corrects the skeletal abnormalities caused by RUNX2 happloinsufficiency [24,25].

Recently, it has been shown that *Twist1* can also inhibit *Atf4* by a direct interaction through the binding to the OSE1 element in the osteocalcin promoter, which further broadens the extensive role of TWIST in the regulation of osteoblast differentiation [26].

MSX1 and MSX2

Muscle segment homeobox or MSX transcription factor was first identified in Drosophila. The *Msx* gene belongs to the family of *Hox* homeogenes, which are critical in early patterning and cell commitment and differentiation. Unlike the other *Hox* genes that are expressed in the axial and appendicular skeleton, *Msx* gene expression is restricted to the head and facial primordial. In humans, at least two *MSX* genes, *MSX1* and *MSX2*, have been identified which are highly expressed during morphogenesis by embryonic tissues that require of epithelial-mesenchymal interactions. A gain-of-function mutation in the *MSX2* gene causes Boston-Type craniosynostosis leading to the premature fusion of calvarial bones that cause abnormal skull shape [27].

In agreement with the human disease pathophysiology, *Msx1* ablation in mice shows abnormal craniofacial development, complete cleft of the secondary palate, impair tooth and alveolar bone development and deformities in several facial and skull bones [28]. These abnormalities lead to early lethality in the knockout mice. MSX2-deficient mice show defects in skull ossification and a persistent calvarial foramen phenotype, due to a defective proliferation of osteoprogenitor cells during skull morphogenesis. Additionally, the null mice also show defects in endochondral bone formation, and abnormal development of teeth, hair follicles, mammary glands and cerebellum [29].

On the other hand, the overexpression of *Msx2* in mice in osteoblasts results in larger calvaria and in an increase in the number of proliferative, early-stage osteoblastic cells, suggesting that MSX2 inhibits osteoblast differentiation and increases the osteoblasts number, albeit in a transient manner [30]. Later, in vitro studies showed that MSX2 directly interacts with RUNX2 and thereby repressing its activity temporarily in the differentiating pre-osteoblasts [31].

In addition to this transient inhibitory activity MSX2 may promote the differentiation of mesenchymal cells into osteoblasts, induced by bone morphogenetic protein 2 (BMP-2) and independent of RUNX2. BMP2 treatment of mesenchymal-like C3H10T1/2 cells resulted in MSX2 expression and in an increase of ALPL activity, while the introduction of MSX2 in these cells resulted in osteogenic differentiation marked by ALPL activity. Interestingly, RUNX2-deficient cells, when treated with BMP2, expressed *Msx2* and *Alpl* indicating that MSX2 map promote osteoblast differentiation independent of RUNX2 [32].

SP7/Osterix

Runx2 expression in the common chondro/osteo progenitors and in late stage chondrocytes implies that a more specific transcription factor must regulate the differentiation of osteoblasts from the progenitor cells. Murine C2C12 myoblasts when treated with BMP2, an osteogenic cytokine, express Type I collagen and Osteocalcin. Nakashima *et al.* used the method of subtraction expression analysis of BMP2-treated and control C2C12 cells to identify a novel osteogenic transcription factor Osterix (OSX) [33].

The murine OSX is a 46kDa protein comprised of 428 amino acids that contains an 85 amino acid zinc finger DNA-binding motif. OSX belonging to the Specificity Protein (SP) family of transcription factors was later named as SP7 [34]. The 'knocking-in' of an IRES-betagalactosidase cassette at a single *Osx* locus in mice showed that OSX is expressed in all developing bones. Mice homozygous for this inactivating mutation died after birth, primarily due to respiratory complications caused by the deformed 'cartilage only' rib cage. Histology and marker gene analysis by *in situ* hybridization showed that skeletal patterning, chondrogenesis and osteoclastogenesis were unaffected in OSX-deficient mice. However, the expression of all osteogenic markers including *Col1a1*, *Bsp* and *Oc* were undetectable in the developing limbs suggesting a total impairment of osteoblast differentiation in the absence of OSX [33].

Nakashima *et al.* showed that there is a complete lack of *Osx* expression in RUNX2-null mice while in *Osx*-null mice, *Runx2* expression was not altered at any embryonic stage. This observation suggested that OSX regulates osteoblast differentiation by acting downstream of RUNX2 [33]. Subsequent studies focussing on the regulatory mechanisms of *Osx* expression confirmed that *Osx* is a direct target for RUNX2. The putative RUNX2 binding site was found in the Osterix promoter and cotransfection experiments using a *Runx2* expression vector and *Osterix* promoter-driven reporter construct in ATDC5 chondrogenic cells showed an upregulation of the *Osx* promoter activity. Furthermore, gel shift assay experiments confirmed that RUNX2 binds directly to the *Osx* promoter [35].

The function of OSX is not restricted to osteoblast differentiation and bone formation during embryonic stages. It is also required for postnatal bone growth and adult bone homeostasis. Since *Osx*-null mice die perinatally, a mouse model for conditional *Osx* knockout was generated using the 'Cre-LoxP' system. Tamoxifen induced Cre recombinase expression and thereby conditional ablation of *Osx* during postnatal stages displayed a reduced new bone formation, decreased *Col1a1, Bsp* and *Oc* RNAs, despite the elevated *Runx2* expression. Additionally, these mutants showed a decreased osteocyte density and a reduced dendrite network in the bone cortex. Interestingly, an excess of mineralized tissue in the long bones of the postnatal mutants was encountered, that was identified as calcified cartilage matrix, which shows that the process of cartilage resorption is severely impaired in these mice, suggesting that this process is tightly coupled to Osterix endochondral bone formation [36]. The same conditional *Osx*-postnatal mutant mice were crossed with Rosa26R reporter mice in order to study the role of Osterix in postnatal stages. Similarly, a reduced mineralized trabecular bone was reported, along with a reduced bone formation rate, suggesting that Osterix inactivation in postnatal stages leads to an osteoblast dysfunction, with no apparent changes in osteoblast proliferation and osteoclastogenesis [37]. Similar results were obtained when the postnatal function of Osterix was assessed through the use of a time-and site specific Cre/loxP system, under the control of the 2.3kb Collagen promoter.

Taking together, these findings propose Osterix as an important regulator of osteoblast function and bone formation in growing and adult bones [38].

β-Catenin

Wnt/β-catenin pathway is involved in many developmental processes including limb patterning and joint formation and also in the regulation of bone mass postnatally. Impaired signalling through this pathway has been linked to familial osteoporosis [39]. In the absence of Wnt, β-catenin is phosphorylated by cytosolic Glycogen synthase kinases (GSK) and eventually degraded by the proteasome machinery. Wnt signalling prevents the phosphorylation of β-catenin leading to its translocation and accumulation inside the nucleus where it interacts with members of the Lef/Tcf transcription factors to activate the target genes. The deletion of GSK phosphorylation sites in β-catenin in osteoblasts results in an osteopetrosis phenotype in mice. This phenotype is caused by an upregulation of Wnt target gene *Osteoprotegerin*, which in turn results in the sequestration of RANKL and impaired osteoclast differentiation. A novel link between OSX and Wnt signaling has been proposed recently. *Dkk1*, a negative regulator of Wnt/β-catenin-signalling pathway has been shown to be a downstream target of *Osx*. In *Osx*-null calvarial cells, no expression of the inhibitor *Dkk1* was detected, and in contrast, several Wnt target genes were overexpressed in these cells [40].

ATF4

Activating transcription factor 4 (ATF4) belongs to the cAMP response element binding (CREB) family of transcription factors. ATF4, also known as CREB2, is required for osteoblast differentiation and function. The ATF4-deficient 13.5 embryos do not have any difference with the WT embryos, which suggest that ATF4 is not essential for early stages of development. However, the expression of Bone sialoprotein and Osteocalcin is delayed in the developing long bones, whereas the expressions of genes characteristic of early osteblastogenesis, such as *Runx2*, *Osx* and *Col1a1* remain unaffected. This altered expression profile of late osteoblast markers suggests that ATF4 is required for the terminal differentiation of osteoblasts.

An important observation, that the trabecular bone is abnormally thin in *Atf4*-null mice lead to a significant finding that the mutant osteoblasts show a defect in Type I collagen synthesis. Interestingly, there was no decrease of *Col1a1* transcripts in these cells, thus, the reduced Type I collagen synthesis was attributed to an impaired amino acid import, a function that is overtly regulated by ATF4 [41]. In RUNX2-deficient cells, no ATF4 was detected, which suggest that ATF4 expression in osteoblasts is dependent on RUNX2 function. Further experiments revealed that Osteocalcin is a target gene for ATF4 which binds to the OSE1 *cis*-acting elements present in the Osteocalcin promoter [41]. The mutational analysis of OSE1 and OSE2 (RUNX2 binding element) demonstrated that both ATF4 and RUNX2 are required for normal osteocalcin expression in osteoblasts. In absence of OSE1 the expression of osteocalcin was markedly reduced while the expression of ATF4 alone was unable to express Osteocalcin mRNA in non-osteoblastic cells that lacked detectable RUNX2 [42].

Atf4 mRNA has been detected in many non-osteoblastic cell types in a comparable amount to that of osteoblasts although ATF4 protein was detected only in the latter. This observation suggests that a complex post-translational process controls the cell type specificity of ATF4. Such a process includes proteasomal degradation of ATF4 in non-osteoblastic cells. Additionally, *Atf4* overexpression in non-osteoblastic cells was able to induce endogenous Osteocalcin expression, property that is also present in the mayor transcription factors that regulate osteoblast differentiation, RUNX2 and OSX [43].

It was shown *in vivo* that ATF4 is a target for ribosomal serine/threonine kinase2 (RSK2). ATF4 phosphorylation is affected in *Rsk2*-null mice which show similar bone phenotype as reported in *Atf4* null mice. Furthermore, it has been shown that Neurofibromin1 (NF1) that regulates RSK2-mediated phosphorylation of ATF4 may act as a negative modulator of ATF4-regulated downstream events. *Nf1* is highly expressed in osteoblasts and mice with ablation of *Nf1* show a complex phenotype that includes an increased bone mass, increase of unmineralized bone matrix and bone resorption [44]. ATF4 is also regulated through a Factor-Inhibiting ATF4-mediated transcription (FIAT), a 66-kD leucine zipper nuclear protein. FIAT interacts with ATF4 and prevents its binding to the OSE1 element in the Osteocalcin promoter. Transgenic mice that overexpress FIAT under the osteoblast-specific *Col1a1* promoter, show a osteopenic phenotype with a decreased bone mineral density and trabecular volume and a reduced mineral apposition and bone formation rates. Unaltered osteoblast proliferation and apoptosis and normal *Runx2, Osterix* and *Atf4* gene expression in these transgenic mice, suggested that osteoblast activity was affected. Osteocalcin transcription was also affected [45]. On the other hand, in cells were FIAT was knocked-down, enhanced mineralization activity could be assessed, with a marked increase in collagen protein secretion [46]. Taken together, these data is in agreement with the suggested role of FIAT as a modulator of ATF4 activity and osteoblast function.

The bone forming cells, osteoblasts; are also involved in the control of endocrine functions in vivo and ATF4 seems to play a major role in this process. ATF4 regulates the expression of *Esp* (Embryonic Stem Cell Phosphatase) a gene that in turn regulates the post-translational carboxylation of Osteocalcin. Under-carboxylated Osteocalcin promotes insulin secretion and insulin sensitivity of different organs and tissues such as liver, muscle and fat. The ATF4-deficient mice show smaller fat pads and low blood glucose levels secondary to an increase in the circulating insulin levels. This data adds to the mechanism of osteoblast-mediated regulation of energy metabolism in the body [47].

Recently, a role for ATF4 in bone resorbing osteoclasts has been proposed. Immunohistoquemical staining showed a strong ATF4 signal in the osteoclast cytoplasm in a mouse monocyte/macrophage cell line. A dramatically reduced TRAP activity was detected in *Atf4*-null bones while in transgenic mice, that overexpress *Atf4* driven by an osteoclast-specific *Trap* promoter, resulted in a severe osteopenic phenotype. There was an upregulation of all the osteoclastic differentiation markers (*Trap, Rank, CatK and Mmp9*) and an increase of bone resorption [48]. ATF4 expression has also been detected in chondrocytes. *Col2a1* promoter driven *Atf4* expression was shown to prevent the bone abnormalities seen in *Atf4*-null mice. This observation suggests that ATF4 in chondrocytes may modulate osteoblast differentiation and function through humoral means [49].

FoxO1

Forkhead box O1 (FOXO1) is a member of the family of ubiquitous transcription factors FoxOs. These transcription factors are activated in order to counteract the effects of Reactive Oxygen Species (ROS). FoxO1 is the main regulator of redox balance in osteoblasts and consequently, controls the bone mass. Cell culture experiments also suggested that FOXO1 plays a role in osteoblast differentiation, since the knocking-down of *FoxO1* in pre-osteoblastic cells showed a reduction in the number of mineralized nodules, together with a significant reduction in RUNX2, Type I collagen, Osteocalcin and MMP13 [50]. Mice lacking *FoxO1* specifically in the osteoblasts showed a low bone mass, decreased bone formation rate and osteoblast numbers. There was a decreased expression of Osterix and a decreased of Type I collagen protein level. FOXO1 has been shown to interact with ATF4 and appear to be a major regulator of ATF4 function in bone [51]. FOXO1 has also been identified as a negative regulator of energy metabolism. It negatively regulates the insulin sensitivity in β-cells, hepatocytes and adipocytes, together with the regulation of β-cell proliferation and hepatic glucose production. This control of energy metabolism is in part carried out by the *FoxO1* expression in osteoblasts, which activates two regulatory mechanisms: firstly, the stimulation of Osteocalcin expression and thereby enhancing β-cell proliferation, insulin secretion and energy expenditure and, secondly, through inhibition of *Esp* expression, and thereby promoting Osteocalcin decarboxylation [52].

B. Diseases Associated with Osteogenic Transcription Factors

Cleidocranial Dysplasia (CCD)

A mutation in the *RUNX2* gene causes a common autosomal dominant skeletal dysplasia called cleidocranial dysplasia. The mutation has been mapped to chromosome 6p21 which results in a substitution of highly conserved amino acids in the DNA-binding domain preventing the binding of RUNX2 to its target sequence [53-55].

The pathognomonic symptoms of CCD have been identified as delayed ossification of the fontanelles and aplasia or hypoplasia of one or both clavicles [56]. The prevalence of CCD among the population is one per million, even though an under-diagnosis can be present given the relative lack of medical complications when compared with other skeletal dysplasias. CCD has been diagnosed in all ethnic groups without any gender predilection.

Among the clinical manifestations of patients with CCD, short stature is common in males and females, but is not enough significant to consider CCD as a dwarfing condition. Some skeletal traces are genua valga, pes planus, hipermobile shoulders and scoliosis. There is no major difference regarding bone fractures among CCD patients and controls. Additionally, join laxity and pain, elbow and knee dislocations, short digits and small hands and feet have been reported. As a consequence of midface hypoplasia and underdeveloped sinuses, upper respiratory complications, recurrent otitis media, ear infections and hearing loss are common. The CCD patients show the same motor and intellectual development as controls as well as pregnancy in females, even though they tend to have more Cesarean section deliveries.

Dental abnormalities are a well-known manifestation in CCD patient, and often are the first clinical sign that leads to CCD diagnosis. Malocclusion is commonly found, whereas supernumerary teeth and impacted teeth are a common cause of surgical interventions, and represent the main cause of treatment in CCD patients [57]. Additionally, a study showed that CCD patients have an increased prevalence of submucous cleft palate over the general population [58].

Saethre Chotzen Syndrome (SCS)

Mutations or deletions in the *TWIST* gene, in the chromosome 7p21-p22 in humans, leads to Saethre-Chotzen syndrome, also known as Acrocephalosyndactyly Type III. SCS is an autosomal dominant disorder with a complete penetrance and variable expressivity that shows a birth prevalence of 1/25.000 to 1/50.000. It is mainly characterized by facial and limb abnormalities and craniosynostosis, the premature fusion of calvarial bones that leads to an abnormal head shape [59, 60]. Among the facial dimorphisms the most prominent features are asymmetry, hypertelorism and maxillary hypoplasia. Other characteristics such as low frontal hairline, strabismus, ptosis of eyelids, abnormal nasal septum, malocclusion, cleft palate and enamel hypoplasia are less recurrent [60]. Microtia, cognitive and learning disabilities, hearing loss, anatomical abnormalities of the middle ear have also been described in patients with SCS [59]. The most common limb abnormalities seen in these patients are syndactyty, polydactyly, brachydactyly and clinodactyly.

Commonly, a surgical management is required in order to treat the craniosynostosis. The cranioplasty consist in the release of the prematurely fused sutures, which includes reposition and reconstruction of the calvaria, such as intracranial fronto-orbital advancement and cranial vault remodelling, which in general have an acceptable aesthetic outcome. Also, some patients may also require midface or ortognatic surgery, in order to correct malocclusions, cleft palate, swallowing or respiratory problems [61, 62].

Boston-Type Craniosynostosis

Boston-Type craniosynostosis is a highly penetrant autosomal dominant genetic disorder caused by a missense mutation in the *MSX2* gene in the human chromosome 5q 35; that is characterized, as all others craniosynostosis, by the premature fusion of calvarial bones with the subsequent abnormality in skull shape [27, 63, 64].

Non-Collagenous Osteogenesis Imperfecta Caused by *SP7/OSX* Mutation

Osteogenesis imperfecta (OI) is a bone-related disorder where in the majority of the cases, the genes encoding for Type I collagen (*COL1A1* and *COL2A1*) are mutated. However, some forms of OI are not associated with any mutation of collagen genes. Recently, in an Egyptian family with a boy with recessive OI, a homozygous single base pair deletion in the

SP7/OSX gene was identified. Clinical assessment showed frequent fractures following minor trauma (6-7 fractures per year), delayed motor milestones, mild asymmetry of the face with prominent forehead, midface hypoplasia, depressed nasal bridge, micrognatia and delayed tooth eruption. Also limbs deformities, scoliosis and short stature were identified and further examination of the patient revealed generalized osteoporosis. The recognition of a mutation in the *SP7/OSX* gene in this case of osteogenesis imperfecta revealed the first human disease related with a mutation in the gene that encodes for the Osterix transcription factor [65].

Coffin-Lowry Syndrome (CLS)

Coffin-Lowry syndrome is a rare, X-linked semidominant syndrome caused by a heterogeneous loss-of-function mutation in the human *RSK2* gene in the chromosome Xp22.2 and presents an estimated incidence of 1:50.000 to 1:100.000 [66, 67]. CLS is classically characterized by mental and growth retardation, facial dysmorphism and digit abnormalities. At birth, affected males show hypotonia and hyperlaxity of joints, hypertelorism and thick lips, which become more protruded with time. Growth retardation and delayed psychomotor development also increase gradually. By adulthood, the CLS patients conserve their marked facial features, and develop dental and skeletal characteristics such as narrow palate, hypodontia, peg-shaped incisors and premature exfoliation of primary teeth [68]. The hands of CLS patients show hyperlaxitude, lax skin and joints and tapering stubby fingers. Among the skeletal abnormalities, the CLS patients show delayed bone development, scoliosis, cranial hyperostosis, delayed bone age and shorter distal phalanges. The variability in mental retardation and cognitive deficiencies among male CLS patients is large but often severe. Additionally it has been reported epilepsy and hearing loss. The carrier females show a highly variable CLS trace, from short digits with normal appearance and intelligence, to moderate facial abnormalities and mental retardation. Obesity and psychiatric diseases have also been reported [67].

Neurofibromatosis Type I

Neurofibromatosis Type1 (NF1) is a genetic autosomal dominant disease caused by a mutation in the *NF1* gene located in chromosome 17q11.2 in humans. It is also called Recklinghausen's disease and has a very specific cutaneous phenotype. The most distinct symptom is the development of neurofibromas around peripheral nerves. Also, the NF1 patients show hyperpigmented macules called café-au-lait, as well as pigmented hamartomas of the iris [69].

Conclusion

The recent advent of molecular genetics and the availability of transgenic and 'knockout' mouse models have immensely contributed to our understanding of osteoblastogenesis. Many of the signalling molecules and the downstream transcription factors that regulate the differentiation of multipotent mesenchymal stem cells to osteoblasts are now well characterized. Every so often researchers in the field are adding new pieces to the complex puzzle of transcriptional regulation of osteoblast differentiation and a more complete picture of how these factors interact with each other and their relative hierarchy in regulating marker gene expression have started to emerge. Since the major transcription factors that regulate the transition of various stages of differentiating osteoblasts have already been identified, the tasks ahead include how these transcription factors may affect each other's function in a spatio-temporal manner. Generation of novel mouse models using more advanced genetic tools e.g. inducible 'knockout', 'knockdown' and over-/miss-expression of target genes may provide important clues in this regard.

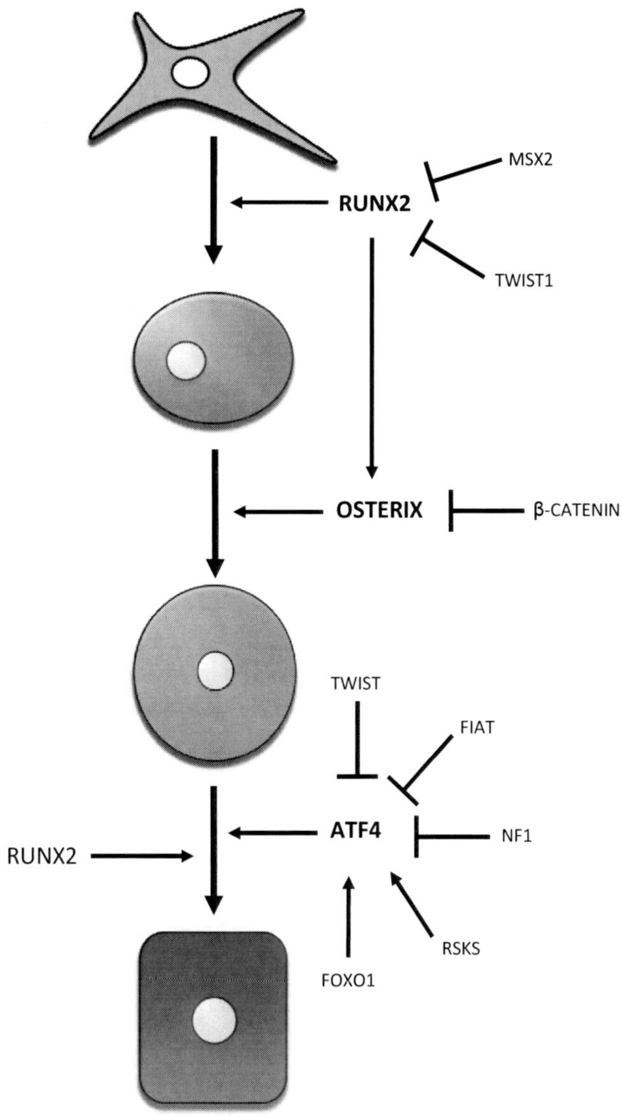

Figure 1. Diagram showing the stages of a differentiating osteoblast and the major transcription factors involved at that stage. The arrows indicate induction of a transcription factor and the perpendicular lines represent negative regulation.

References

[1] Ducy P, Karsenty G. Two distinct osteoblast-specific cis-acting elements control expression of a mouse osteocalcin gene. *Molecular and cellular biology.* 1995;15(4):1858-69. Epub 1995/04/01.

[2] Pepling ME, Gergen JP. Conservation and function of the transcriptional regulatory protein Runt. *Proceedings of the National Academy of Sciences of the United States of America.* 1995;92(20):9087-91. Epub 1995/09/26.

[3] Geoffroy V, Ducy P, Karsenty G. A PEBP2 alpha/AML-1-related factor increases osteocalcin promoter activity through its binding to an osteoblast-specific cis-acting element. *The Journal of biological chemistry.* 1995;270(52):30973-9. Epub 1995/12/29.

[4] Ducy P, Zhang R, Geoffroy V, Ridall AL, Karsenty G. Osf2/Cbfa1: a transcriptional activator of osteoblast differentiation. *Cell.* 1997;89(5):747-54. Epub 1997/05/30.

[5] Kim IS, Otto F, Zabel B, Mundlos S. Regulation of chondrocyte differentiation by Cbfa1. *Mechanisms of development.* 1999;80(2):159-70. Epub 1999/03/12.

[6] Sudhakar S, Li Y, Katz MS, Elango N. Translational regulation is a control point in RUNX2/Cbfa1 gene expression. *Biochemical and biophysical research communications.* 2001;289(2):616-22. Epub 2001/11/22.

[7] Harada H, Tagashira S, Fujiwara M, Ogawa S, Katsumata T, Yamaguchi A, et al. Cbfa1 isoforms exert functional differences in osteoblast differentiation. *The Journal of biological chemistry.* 1999;274(11):6972-8. Epub 1999/03/06.

[8] Thirunavukkarasu K, Mahajan M, McLarren KW, Stifani S, Karsenty G. Two domains unique to osteoblast-specific transcription factor Osf2/Cbfa1 contribute to its transactivation function and its inability to heterodimerize with Cbfbeta. *Molecular and cellular biology.* 1998;18(7):4197-208. Epub 1998/06/25.

[9] Gerstenfeld LC, Cruceta J, Shea CM, Sampath K, Barnes GL, Einhorn TA. Chondrocytes provide morphogenic signals that selectively induce osteogenic differentiation of mesenchymal stem cells. *Journal of bone and mineral research : the official journal of the American Society for Bone and Mineral Research.* 2002;17(2):221-30. Epub 2002/01/29.

[10] Komori T, Yagi H, Nomura S, Yamaguchi A, Sasaki K, Deguchi K, et al. Targeted disruption of Cbfa1 results in a complete lack of bone formation owing to maturational arrest of osteoblasts. *Cell.* 1997;89(5):755-64. Epub 1997/05/30.

[11] Otto F, Thornell AP, Crompton T, Denzel A, Gilmour KC, Rosewell IR, et al. Cbfa1, a candidate gene for cleidocranial dysplasia syndrome, is essential for osteoblast differentiation and bone development. *Cell.* 1997;89(5):765-71. Epub 1997/05/30.

[12] Inada M, Yasui T, Nomura S, Miyake S, Deguchi K, Himeno M, et al. Maturational disturbance of chondrocytes in Cbfa1-deficient mice. Developmental dynamics : *an official publication of the American Association of Anatomists.* 1999;214(4):279-90. Epub 1999/04/23.

[13] Lengner CJ, Drissi H, Choi JY, van Wijnen AJ, Stein JL, Stein GS, et al. Activation of the bone-related Runx2/Cbfa1 promoter in mesenchymal condensations and developing chondrocytes of the axial skeleton. *Mechanisms of development.* 2002;114(1-2):167-70. Epub 2002/08/15.

[14] Takeda S, Bonnamy JP, Owen MJ, Ducy P, Karsenty G. Continuous expression of Cbfa1 in nonhypertrophic chondrocytes uncovers its ability to induce hypertrophic chondrocyte differentiation and partially rescues Cbfa1-deficient mice. *Genes and development*. 2001;15(4):467-81. Epub 2001/03/07.

[15] Stricker S, Fundele R, Vortkamp A, Mundlos S. Role of Runx genes in chondrocyte differentiation. *Developmental biology*. 2002;245(1):95-108. Epub 2002/04/24.

[16] Himeno M, Enomoto H, Liu W, Ishizeki K, Nomura S, Kitamura Y, et al. Impaired vascular invasion of Cbfa1-deficient cartilage engrafted in the spleen. *Journal of bone and mineral research : the official journal of the American Society for Bone and Mineral Research*. 2002;17(7):1297-305. Epub 2002/07/05.

[17] Ducy P, Starbuck M, Priemel M, Shen J, Pinero G, Geoffroy V, et al. A Cbfa1-dependent genetic pathway controls bone formation beyond embryonic development. *Genes and development*. 1999;13(8):1025-36. Epub 1999/04/24.

[18] Tsuji K, Komori T, Noda M. Aged mice require full transcription factor, Runx2/Cbfa1, gene dosage for cancellous bone regeneration after bone marrow ablation. *Journal of bone and mineral research : the official journal of the American Society for Bone and Mineral Research*. 2004;19(9):1481-9. Epub 2004/08/18.

[19] Geoffroy V, Kneissel M, Fournier B, Boyde A, Matthias P. High bone resorption in adult aging transgenic mice overexpressing cbfa1/runx2 in cells of the osteoblastic lineage. *Molecular and cellular biology*. 2002;22(17):6222-33. Epub 2002/08/09.

[20] Thisse B, Stoetzel C, Gorostiza-Thisse C, Perrin-Schmitt F. Sequence of the twist gene and nuclear localization of its protein in endomesodermal cells of early Drosophila embryos. *The EMBO journal*. 1988;7(7):2175-83. Epub 1988/07/01.

[21] Chen ZF, Behringer RR. twist is required in head mesenchyme for cranial neural tube morphogenesis. *Genes and development*. 1995;9(6):686-99. Epub 1995/03/15.

[22] Lee MS, Lowe GN, Strong DD, Wergedal JE, Glackin CA. TWIST, a basic helix-loop-helix transcription factor, can regulate the human osteogenic lineage. *Journal of cellular biochemistry*. 1999;75(4):566-77. Epub 1999/11/26.

[23] Isenmann S, Arthur A, Zannettino AC, Turner JL, Shi S, Glackin CA, et al. TWIST family of basic helix-loop-helix transcription factors mediate human mesenchymal stem cell growth and commitment. *Stem cells*. 2009;27(10):2457-68. Epub 2009/07/18.

[24] Bialek P, Kern B, Yang X, Schrock M, Sosic D, Hong N, et al. A twist code determines the onset of osteoblast differentiation. *Developmental cell*. 2004;6(3):423-35. Epub 2004/03/20.

[25] Yousfi M, Lasmoles F, Marie PJ. TWIST inactivation reduces CBFA1/RUNX2 expression and DNA binding to the osteocalcin promoter in osteoblasts. *Biochemical and biophysical research communications*. 2002;297(3):641-4. Epub 2002/09/25.

[26] Danciu TE, Li Y, Koh A, Xiao G, McCauley LK, Franceschi RT. The basic helix loop helix transcription factor Twist1 is a novel regulator of ATF4 in osteoblasts. *Journal of cellular biochemistry*. 2012;113(1):70-9. Epub 2011/08/26.

[27] Jabs EW, Muller U, Li X, Ma L, Luo W, Haworth IS, et al. A mutation in the homeodomain of the human MSX2 gene in a family affected with autosomal dominant craniosynostosis. *Cell*. 1993;75(3):443-50. Epub 1993/11/05.

[28] Satokata I, Maas R. Msx1 deficient mice exhibit cleft palate and abnormalities of craniofacial and tooth development. *Nature genetics*. 1994;6(4):348-56. Epub 1994/04/01.

[29] Satokata I, Ma L, Ohshima H, Bei M, Woo I, Nishizawa K, et al. Msx2 deficiency in mice causes pleiotropic defects in bone growth and ectodermal organ formation. *Nature genetics*. 2000;24(4):391-5. Epub 2000/03/31.

[30] Liu YH, Tang Z, Kundu RK, Wu L, Luo W, Zhu D, et al. Msx2 gene dosage influences the number of proliferative osteogenic cells in growth centers of the developing murine skull: a possible mechanism for MSX2-mediated craniosynostosis in humans. *Developmental biology*. 1999;205(2):260-74. Epub 1999/01/26.

[31] Shirakabe K, Terasawa K, Miyama K, Shibuya H, Nishida E. Regulation of the activity of the transcription factor Runx2 by two homeobox proteins, Msx2 and Dlx5. *Genes to cells : devoted to molecular and cellular mechanisms*. 2001;6(10):851-6. Epub 2001/10/31.

[32] Ichida F, Nishimura R, Hata K, Matsubara T, Ikeda F, Hisada K, et al. Reciprocal roles of MSX2 in regulation of osteoblast and adipocyte differentiation. *The Journal of biological chemistry*. 2004;279(32):34015-22. Epub 2004/06/04.

[33] Nakashima K, Zhou X, Kunkel G, Zhang Z, Deng JM, Behringer RR, et al. The novel zinc finger-containing transcription factor osterix is required for osteoblast differentiation and bone formation. *Cell*. 2002;108(1):17-29. Epub 2002/01/17.

[34] Gao Y, Jheon A, Nourkeyhani H, Kobayashi H, Ganss B. Molecular cloning, structure, expression, and chromosomal localization of the human Osterix (SP7) gene. Gene. 2004;341:101-10. Epub 2004/10/12.

[35] Nishio Y, Dong Y, Paris M, O'Keefe RJ, Schwarz EM, Drissi H. Runx2-mediated regulation of the zinc finger Osterix/Sp7 gene. *Gene*. 2006;372:62-70. Epub 2006/04/01.

[36] Zhou X, Zhang Z, Feng JQ, Dusevich VM, Sinha K, Zhang H, et al. Multiple functions of Osterix are required for bone growth and homeostasis in postnatal mice. *Proceedings of the National Academy of Sciences of the United States of America*. 2010;107(29):12919-24. Epub 2010/07/10.

[37] Baek WY, de Crombrugghe B, Kim JE. Postnatally induced inactivation of Osterix in osteoblasts results in the reduction of bone formation and maintenance. *Bone*. 2010;46(4):920-8. Epub 2009/12/23.

[38] Baek WY, Lee MA, Jung JW, Kim SY, Akiyama H, de Crombrugghe B, et al. Positive regulation of adult bone formation by osteoblast-specific transcription factor osterix. Journal of bone and mineral research *: the official journal of the American Society for Bone and Mineral Research*. 2009;24(6):1055-65. Epub 2008/12/31.

[39] Pinson KI, Brennan J, Monkley S, Avery BJ, Skarnes WC. An LDL-receptor-related protein mediates Wnt signalling in mice. *Nature*. 2000;407(6803):535-8. Epub 2000/10/12.

[40] Zhang C, Cho K, Huang Y, Lyons JP, Zhou X, Sinha K, et al. Inhibition of Wnt signaling by the osteoblast-specific transcription factor Osterix. *Proceedings of the National Academy of Sciences of the United States of America*. 2008;105(19):6936-41. Epub 2008/05/07.

[41] Yang X, Matsuda K, Bialek P, Jacquot S, Masuoka HC, Schinke T, et al. ATF4 is a substrate of RSK2 and an essential regulator of osteoblast biology; implication for Coffin-Lowry Syndrome. *Cell*. 2004;117(3):387-98. Epub 2004/04/28.

[42] Xiao G, Jiang D, Ge C, Zhao Z, Lai Y, Boules H, et al. Cooperative interactions between activating transcription factor 4 and Runx2/Cbfa1 stimulate osteoblast-specific

osteocalcin gene expression. *The Journal of biological chemistry*. 2005;280(35):30689-96. Epub 2005/07/08.

[43] Yang X, Karsenty G. ATF4, the osteoblast accumulation of which is determined post-translationally, can induce osteoblast-specific gene expression in non-osteoblastic cells. *The Journal of biological chemistry*. 2004;279(45):47109-14. Epub 2004/09/21.

[44] Elefteriou F, Benson MD, Sowa H, Starbuck M, Liu X, Ron D, et al. ATF4 mediation of NF1 functions in osteoblast reveals a nutritional basis for congenital skeletal dysplasiae. *Cell metabolism*. 2006;4(6):441-51. Epub 2006/12/05.

[45] Yu VW, Ambartsoumian G, Verlinden L, Moir JM, Prud'homme J, Gauthier C, et al. FIAT represses ATF4-mediated transcription to regulate bone mass in transgenic mice. *The Journal of cell biology*. 2005;169(4):591-601. Epub 2005/05/25.

[46] Yu VW, El-Hoss J, St-Arnaud R. FIAT inhibition increases osteoblast activity by modulating Atf4-dependent functions. *Journal of cellular biochemistry*. 2009;106(1):186-92. Epub 2008/11/19.

[47] Yoshizawa T, Hinoi E, Jung DY, Kajimura D, Ferron M, Seo J, et al. The transcription factor ATF4 regulates glucose metabolism in mice through its expression in osteoblasts. *The Journal of clinical investigation*. 2009;119(9):2807-17. Epub 2009/09/04.

[48] Cao H, Yu S, Yao Z, Galson DL, Jiang Y, Zhang X, et al. Activating transcription factor 4 regulates osteoclast differentiation in mice. *The Journal of clinical investigation*. 2010;120(8):2755-66. Epub 2010/07/16.

[49] Wang W, Lian N, Ma Y, Li L, Gallant RC, Elefteriou F, et al. Chondrocytic Atf4 regulates osteoblast differentiation and function via Ihh. *Development*. 2012;139(3):601-11. Epub 2011/12/23.

[50] Siqueira MF, Flowers S, Bhattacharya R, Faibish D, Behl Y, Kotton DN, et al. FOXO1 modulates osteoblast differentiation. *Bone*. 2011;48(5):1043-51. Epub 2011/02/02.

[51] Rached MT, Kode A, Xu L, Yoshikawa Y, Paik JH, Depinho RA, et al. FoxO1 is a positive regulator of bone formation by favoring protein synthesis and resistance to oxidative stress in osteoblasts. *Cell metabolism*. 2010;11(2):147-60. Epub 2010/02/10.

[52] Rached MT, Kode A, Silva BC, Jung DY, Gray S, Ong H, et al. FoxO1 expression in osteoblasts regulates glucose homeostasis through regulation of osteocalcin in mice. *The Journal of clinical investigation*. 2010;120(1):357-68. Epub 2009/12/30.

[53] Lee B, Thirunavukkarasu K, Zhou L, Pastore L, Baldini A, Hecht J, et al. Missense mutations abolishing DNA binding of the osteoblast-specific transcription factor OSF2/CBFA1 in cleidocranial dysplasia. *Nature genetics*. 1997;16(3):307-10. Epub 1997/07/01.

[54] Zhang YW, Bae SC, Takahashi E, Ito Y. The cDNA cloning of the transcripts of human PEBP2alphaA/CBFA1 mapped to 6p12.3-p21.1, the locus for cleidocranial dysplasia. *Oncogene*. 1997;15(3):367-71. Epub 1997/07/17.

[55] Mundlos S. Cleidocranial dysplasia: clinical and molecular genetics. *Journal of medical genetics*. 1999;36(3):177-82. Epub 1999/04/16.

[56] Shen Z, Zou CC, Yang RW, Zhao ZY. Cleidocranial dysplasia: report of 3 cases and literature review. *Clinical pediatrics*. 2009;48(2):194-8. Epub 2008/10/04.

[57] Bufalino A, Paranaiba LM, Gouvea AF, Gueiros LA, Martelli-Junior H, Junior JJ, et al. Cleidocranial dysplasia: oral features and genetic analysis of 11 patients. *Oral diseases*. 2012;18(2):184-90. Epub 2011/10/26.

[58] Cooper SC, Flaitz CM, Johnston DA, Lee B, Hecht JT. A natural history of cleidocranial dysplasia. *American journal of medical genetics.* 2001;104(1):1-6. Epub 2001/12/18.

[59] Lamonica DA, Maximino LP, Feniman MR, Silva GK, Zanchetta S, Abramides DV, et al. Saethre-Chotzen Syndrome, Pro136His TWIST Mutation, Hearing Loss, and External and Middle Ear Structural Anomalies: Report on a Brazilian Family. *The Cleft palate-craniofacial journal* : official publication of the American Cleft Palate-Craniofacial Association. 2010;47(5):548-52. Epub 2010/02/27.

[60] Howard TD, Paznekas WA, Green ED, Chiang LC, Ma N, Ortiz de Luna RI, et al. Mutations in TWIST, a basic helix-loop-helix transcription factor, in Saethre-Chotzen syndrome. *Nature genetics.* 1997;15(1):36-41. Epub 1997/01/01.

[61] Foo R, Guo Y, McDonald-McGinn DM, Zackai EH, Whitaker LA, Bartlett SP. The natural history of patients treated for TWIST1-confirmed Saethre-Chotzen syndrome. *Plastic and reconstructive surgery.* 2009;124(6):2085-95. Epub 2009/12/03.

[62] Stoler JM, Rogers GF, Mulliken JB. The frequency of palatal anomalies in Saethre-Chotzen syndrome. *The Cleft palate-craniofacial journal* : official publication of the American Cleft Palate-Craniofacial Association. 2009;46(3):280-4. Epub 2009/08/01.

[63] Ma L, Golden S, Wu L, Maxson R. The molecular basis of Boston-type craniosynostosis: the Pro148-->His mutation in the N-terminal arm of the MSX2 homeodomain stabilizes DNA binding without altering nucleotide sequence preferences. *Human molecular genetics.* 1996;5(12):1915-20. Epub 1996/12/01.

[64] Bernardini L, Castori M, Capalbo A, Mokini V, Mingarelli R, Simi P, et al. Syndromic craniosynostosis due to complex chromosome 5 rearrangement and MSX2 gene triplication. *American journal of medical genetics Part A.* 2007;143A(24):2937-43. Epub 2007/11/15.

[65] Lapunzina P, Aglan M, Temtamy S, Caparros-Martin JA, Valencia M, Leton R, et al. Identification of a frameshift mutation in Osterix in a patient with recessive osteogenesis imperfecta. *American journal of human genetics.* 2010;87(1):110-4. Epub 2010/06/29.

[66] Biancalana V, Briard ML, David A, Gilgenkrantz S, Kaplan J, Mathieu M, et al. Confirmation and refinement of the genetic localization of the Coffin-Lowry syndrome locus in Xp22.1-p22.2. *American journal of human genetics.* 1992;50(5):981-7. Epub 1992/05/01.

[67] Pereira PM, Schneider A, Pannetier S, Heron D, Hanauer A. Coffin-Lowry syndrome. *European journal of human genetics* : EJHG. 2010;18(6):627-33. Epub 2009/11/06.

[68] Igari K, Hozumi Y, Monma Y, Mayanagi H. A case of Coffin-Lowry syndrome with premature exfoliation of primary teeth. International journal of paediatric dentistry / the British Paedodontic Society [and] the *International Association of Dentistry for Children.* 2006;16(3):213-7. Epub 2006/04/29.

[69] Gerber PA, Antal AS, Neumann NJ, Homey B, Matuschek C, Peiper M, et al. Neurofibromatosis. *European journal of medical research.* 2009;14(3):102-5. Epub 2009/04/22.

In: Osteoblasts
Editor: Hugo Scheurer

ISBN: 978-1-62417-806-1

Chapter 5

BMP and Osteoblastogenesis Inhibitors

Shoichiro Kokabu*
Department of Developmental Biology, Harvard School
of Dental Medicine, Boston, Massachusetts, US

Abstract

Bone morphogenetic proteins (BMPs) were originally discovered as factors that induce ectopic bone formation when implanted into muscle tissue and that also stimulate osteoblast differentiation of various cell types. BMPs are the most thoroughly studied of the bone regeneration molecules and have received FDA approval for applications related to bone regeneration in humans. However the clinical utility of BMPs is limited by difficulties with optimal delivery, an identification the BMPs target cells involved in bone regeneration, and a lack of understanding of the systems that modulate BMP signaling or osteoblast differentiation.

In this chapter, we will focus on BMP signaling and it's inhibitors in osteoblastogenesis. In addition we will discuss therapeutic prospects of bone related diseases such as osteoporosis and bone tissue engineering of bone by using BMP signaling.

In BMP signaling transduction, the BMP-bound type II receptor phosphorylates the type I receptor. The activated type I receptor, in turn, phosphorylates downstream substrates such as receptor-regulated Smads (R-Smads), including Smad1, Smad5, and Smad8, in addition to mitogen-activated protein kinases (MAPKs) such as Erk, Jnk and p38. Smads play a central role among the downstream signaling effectors of BMP receptors and also plays an important role in osteoblast differentiation.

R-Smads phosphorylated by BMP receptors form heteromeric complexes with Smad4 and directly activate the transcription BMP-responsive genes, which include Id1, Id2 and Id3. Both Osterix (Osx) and Runx2 are master regulators of osteoblast differentiation and are also activated by BMP-Smad signaling.

---

* Corresponding author: Shoichiro Kokabu DDS, PhD. Department of Developmental Biology, Harvard School of Dental Medicine, 188 Longwood Ave, REB513, Boston, MA 02115. Phone: 617/432-5912, Fax: 617/ 432-3246, E-mail: shoichiro_kokabu@hsdm.harvard.edu, r2004038@saitama-med.ac.jp, kokabu2@mac.com, kokabu2@gmail.com.

BMP signaling and BMP-induced osteoblastogenesis, are negatively regulated by various factors including MicroRNAs (miRNAs). BMP antagonists such as Noggin, Chordin, DAN family members, and BMP3 prevent the binding of BMPs to their receptors in the extracellular space. A pseudoreceptor, BAMBI, acts as a dominant-negative receptor for members of the transforming growth factor beta (TGFβ) superfamily on plasma membrane. Repulsive guidance molecule (RGM) b/DRAGON also acts as BMP signal inhibitors on the plasma membrane. Smad6 and Smad7 inhibit the kinase activity of type I receptors by direct interaction in the cytoplasm. Smad ubiquitination regulatory factor 1 (Smurf1), a member of the HECT family of E3 ubiquitin ligases, causes the ubiquitination and degradation of Smad1 and Smad5. Protein phosphatase magnesium-dependent 1A (PPM1A) and Small C-terminal domain phosphatase 1 (SCP1), which have been identified as Smad phosphatases, target unknown substrates thereby suppressing osteoblast differentiation in addition to dephosphorylating phosphorylated Smads. Zinc-finger and RAN-binding domain-containing protein 2 (ZRANB2) bind Smads and inhibit Smad transcriptional activity. Several nuclear factors such as Twist, STAT1, Schnurri3, ZPF521, HES, and p53, interact with Runx2 or Osx thereby suppressing osteoblastogenesis. MicroRNAs (miRNAs) are key post-transcriptional regulators of gene expression. Several miRNAs inhibits osteoblastogenesis to bind to target sequence and negatively regulate gene expression, which are important for osteoblast differentiation.

As just described, numerous inhibitors are involved in osteoblastogenesis. Therefore, a precise understanding and novel methods to remove these inhibitory systems of osteoblastogenesis may shed light on the treatment of bone related diseases or tissue engineering of bone.

Bone Morphogenetic Proteins

Bone morphogenetic proteins (BMPs) were originally discovered and identified as an ectopic bone inducer in bone matrix in 1965. BMPs are now known to be multifunctional factors in vertebarates and invertebrates. Marshall R. Urist (1965) first prepared demineralized bone by treating bone with hydrochloric acid and then implanting the demineralized bone in muscle tissues. A few weeks after transplantation, he found that new cartilage and bone tissues with marrow had been ectopically formed in muscle tissue [1].

This ectopic bone inducer in muscle tissues was subsequently named " bone morphogenetic protein," because it disappeared after trypsin digestion [2]. However, all attempt to isolate and identify BMP were unsuccessful for more than 20 years after Urist's original findings because of the difficulty in isolating BMP from bone matrix. BMP activity was water insoluble and could be extracted from demineralized bone matrix with protein denaturants [2, 3, 4].

In addition, measurement of BMP activity was possible only in an *in vivo* assay system. Since bone-inducing activity was the sole parameter for measurement of BMPs before their molecular cloning, each sample obtained during the process of purification of BMPs had to be implanted in muscle tissues *in vivo* for a few weeks to examine its activity.

Using the peptide sequence information obtained, Wozney et al. (1988) cloned cDNAs for human BMP1-BMP4. BMP1 was a novel metalloproteinase, whereas BMP2, 3, and 4 were distinct but structurally related to one another and were shown to be novel members of the TGFβ superfamily [5].

Wozney et al. (1988) showed that each recombinant BMP protein, including BMP1, induced cartilage or bone formation *in vivo* [5]. Since TGFβ per se failed to induce ectopic bone formation, the bone inducing activity is unique to BMPs within TGFβ superfamily [6].

To date a lot of investigators have attempted to clarify the effect of BMPs on osteoblastogenesis *in vivo* and *in vitro*. Several experiments have shown that BMPs stimulate osteoblast differentiation in various cell types include periosteal cells, muscle satellite cells, vessel pericytes and bone marrow stromal cells [7, 8, 9, 10, 11].

Furthermore, plenty of molecules, which regulate BMP signaling and osteoblastogenesis have been reported.

BMP-Smad Signaling

BMP signaling is transduced by two different types of transmembrane serine/threonine kinase receptors termed type I and II receptors [12, 13]. To date, three type I BMP receptors have been identified; ALK3 (BMPRIA) binds only to BMPs, ALK6 (BMPRIB) binds to BMPs and anti-mullerian hormone (AMH), and ALK2 recognizes BMPs and activin. Type II receptors that exhibit BMP binding are BMPRII, a receptor that recognizes only BMPs, and Acvr2a and Acvr2b that shared by BMPs and activin [14].

The BMP-bound type II receptor phosphorylates the type I receptor. The activated type I receptor, in turn, phosphorylates downstream substrates such as receptor-regulated Smads (R-Smads), including Smad1, Smad5, and Smad8, in addition to mitogen-activated protein kinases (MAPKs) such as Erk, Jnk and p38 [15]. Smads play a central role among the downstream signaling effectors of BMP receptors and also play an important role in osteoblast differentiation [16]. R-Smads phosphorylated by BMP receptors on two serine residues in the Ser-X-Ser (SXS) motif at the C terminus [17, 18, 19]. Phosphorylated R-Smads form heteromeric complexes with Smad4 and directly activates the transcription BMP-responsive genes, which include Id1, Id2 and Id3 [20, 21, 22, 23].

Extracellular Inhibitor

Extracellularly, a larger number of secreted proteins bind to BMPs and prevent their binding to specific receptors. Noggin, chordin, chordin-like1, chordin-like 2, ectodin/uterine sensitization-associated gene-1 (USAG-1), follistatin, Gremlin, Cerberus, and DNA family members have been identified as BMP antagonists in various animal species [24, 12]. Expression of some antagonists such as Noggin and Gremlin are up-regulated by BMPs, which suggests that the antagonists establish a negative feedback loop [25, 26].

BMP3 is regarded as an antagonist of the osteoinductive BMPs. BMP3 is the most abundant BMP in bone matrix and is mainly secreted by osteoblasts and osteocytes [27, 28]. Adult mice lacking BMP3 have increased bone mass while mice with increased BMP3 levels in bone show delayed endochondral ossification with spontaneous rib fractures [27, 29]. Using *in vitro* cultures of primary bone marrow stromal cells, we demonstrated that over-expression of BMP3 suppresses osteoblast differentiation while loss of BMP3 increases colony-forming unit fibroblasts and colony-forming unit osteoblasts. This ability of BMP3 to affect osteoblast differentiation is due to its interaction with Acvr2b since knockdown of endogenous Acvr2b in BMSCs reduced the suppressive effect of BMP3 on osteoblast differentiation [28].

Cytomembrane Inhibitors

At the cell membrane, BAMBI, a pseudo receptor for TGFβ superfamily, which lacks the intracellular domain of the serine-threonine kinase receptors, inhibits ligand-induced signaling by preventing the formation of signaling receptor complexes [30]. The expression of BAMBI is induced by BMP and TGFβ as well as by Wnt/β-catenin signaling [30, 31].

Repulsive guidance molecule (RGM) b/DRAGON, an RGM family members, is secretory a glycosylphosphatidylinositol (GPI)-anchored membrane protein. DRAGON binds to BMP ligands as well as type I and type II BMP receptors thereby enhancing BMP signaling [32]. In contrast, Kanomata et al. (2009) reported that over-expression of DRAGON suppresses the activity of alkaline phosphatase (ALP), which is typical marker of osteoblast differentiation induced by BMPs in C2C12 myoblasts. [33].

Intracellular Inhibitors

Smad6 and Smad7 inhibit the kinase activity of type I receptors by direct interaction in the cytoplasm [34, 35]. Smad ubiquitination regulatory factor 1 (Smurf1), a member of the HECT family of E3 ubiquitin ligases, has been found to interact with Smad1 and Smad5 via the PPAY motif in their linker regions, thereby triggering their ubiquitination and degradation [36]. Smurf2, which is also HECT family of E3 ubiquitin ligases, preferentially targets Smad1 for ubiquitination and proteasome-mediated degradation [37].

Distinct types of phosphatases, small C-terminal domain phosphatases 1(SCP1) and protein phosphatase magnesium-dependent 1A (PPM1A), have been identified as enzymes that stimulate the dephosphorylation of Smads [38, 39, 40]. SCP1 and PPM1A suppress BMP activity by dephosphorylating the C-terminal SXS motifs in Smad proteins [38, 40].

To determine the role of the phosphorylation and dephosphorylation of Smad1, we used a constitutively active Smad1 mutant expression plasmid, Smad1 (DVD), in which the C-terminal serine residues have been substituted by aspartic acids [16].

This Smad1 mutant, Smad1 (DVD), is able to induce ALP activity without the use of BMP ligands or BMP receptors in C2C12 cells. SCP1 and PPM1A suppress ALP activity induced by Smad1 (DVD) even though Smad1 (DVD) lacks the C-term SCP1 and PPM1A serine motifs. From experiments of phosphatase activity-deficient mutants, the inhibitory effect of PPM1A and SCP1 on BMP-induced osteoblast differentiation is dependent on their phosphatase activities. Moreover, PPM1A over-expression led to a reduction of Smad1 protein levels, which was blocked by Lactacystin, a proteasome inhibitors while SCP1 over-expression suppressed osteoblast differentiation induced by Runx2 over-expression, implying that dephosphorylation of non-Smad targets contribute to the inhibition of the BMP pathway by SCP1 and PPM1A [41, 42].

Zinc-finger and RAN-binding domain-containing protein 2 (ZRANB2) was identified by proteomic analysis as a protein which interacted strongly with Smad1, Smad5, and Smad8 and weakly with Smad4. Over-expression of Zranb2 inhibited BMP-induced osteoblast differentiation in C2C12 *in vitro*, and the injection of Zranb2 mRNA into zebrafish embryos induced dorsalizaition [43].

Tob is a member of the emerging family of antiproliferative proteins. Mice carrying a targeted deletion of the Tob gene have a greater bone mass resulting from increased numbers of osteoblasts. Over-expression of Tob represses BMP2-induced, Smad-mediated transcriptional activation. Tob associates with R-Smads and co-localizes with these Smads in the nuclear bodies upon BMP2 stimulation [44]. Tob also co-localizes with Smad6 at the plasma membrane and enhances the interaction between Smad6 and activated BMP type I receptors. Thus Tob cooperates with Smad6 to inhibit endogenous BMP signaling in cultured mammalian cells (C2C12 and COS7) [45, 44].

Over-expression of Cas-interacting zinc finger protein (CIZ) in MC3T3E1 cells suppresses ALP activity and mRNA levels of osteocalcin and type I collagen induced by BMP2. CIZ over-expression also suppresses BMP2-induced enhancement of the mRNA expression of Runx2. BMP-induced Smad transcriptional activity was blocked by CIZ over-expression. Over-expression of CIZ suppresses the formation of mineralized nodules in osteoblastic cell cultures [46]. Bone volume and bone formation are increased in CIZ-deficient mice, whereas bone resorption is not altered. CIZ deficiency facilitates mRNA levels of ALP and Osx in whole long bones and increases newly formed bone mass after femoral bone marrow ablation *in vivo*. BMP2-induced bone formation on adult mouse calvarial bone *in vivo* was enhanced by CIZ deficiency [47].

Ubc9 (ubiquitin conjugating enzyme 9) is a unique E2-SUMOylation enzyme. siRNA knockdown of Ubc9 enhances osteoblast differentiation induced by BMP2 in C2C12 cells and ST2 cells. Ubc9 knockdown elevates the BMP signaling transduction and reduces the expression of muscle-related genes in cooperation with BMP2 [48].

Nuclear Inhibitors, Which Interact with Runx2 or Osx

Both Osterix (Osx) and Runx2 are master regulators of osteoblast differentiation and are activated by BMP-Smad signaling [49, 50].

Runx2, a Runt domain-containing transcription factor, is indispensable for osteoblast differentiation during both endochondral and intramembranous ossification. Homozygous deletion of Runx2 in mice resulted in a complete lack of osteoblasts [51, 52], while haploinsufficiency of Runx2 in mice or Runx2 in humans led to hypoplastic clavicles and delayed closure of the fontanelles, defects that are characteristic of cleidocranial dysplasia in humans [53, 54]. In addition to being needed for osteoblast differentiation, Runx2 is necessary for the proper function of mature osteoblasts, including the synthesis of bone matrix [55].

Some nuclear factors such as Twist1 [56], Hand2 (heart and neural crest derivatives expressed 2) [57], ZFP521 (zinc-finger protein 521) [58], STAT1 (signal transducer and activator of transcription 1) [59], Schnurri3 [60], Gli3 [61], Hoxa2 [62] and the Hes (Hairy an

Enhancer of Split) and Hey (Hes-related with YRPW motif) protein [63, 64], have been found to suppress Runx2 levels or activity. These factors also use a range of mechanisms, including blocking Runx2 DNA binding, nuclear translocation and protein expression. Finally, Runx2 regulation of target gene expression is likely to be modulated by proteins that govern chromatin modification. For instance, histone deacetylase 4 (HDAC4) was shown to suppress Runx2 function in chondrocytes to inhibit hypertrophy [65]. It remains to be determined whether HDAC4 or a related molecule regulates Runx2 activity in the osteoblast lineage *in vivo*. As described above, SCP1, which is one of the Smads phosphatase, suppresses Runx2-induced osteoblast differentiation in C2C12 cells. However SCP1 did not affect transcriptional activity or protein levels of Runx2, suggested that SCP1 targets the effector of downstream of Runx2 in BMP-Smad-Runx2 axis to suppress osteoblastogenesis [42].

Osx a transcription factor containing three C2H2-type zinc-fingers, is necessary for osteoblast differentiation. Osx was discovered as a BMP-induced gene in C2C12 cells, and its deletion resulted in complete absence of osteoblasts in mouse embryos, despite the relatively normal expression of Runx2 [50]. These results, together with the observation that Osx expression was abolished in Runx2-null mice, indicate that Osx functions down stream of Runx2 during osteoblast differentiation.

In contrast to Runx2 deletion, which leads to a hypoplastic perichondrium, loss of Osx results in ectopic cartilage formation beneath a thickened perichondrium at the diaphysis (where a bone collar normally forms), presumably owing to a fate switch of progenitors to chondrocytes instead of osteoblasts [50]. Beyond its role in differentiation during embryogenesis, Osx is crucial for postnatal osteoblast and osteocyte differentiation and function [66].

Thus, Osx has important roles at multiple stages within the osteoblast lineage, both during embryonic development and in postnatal life. Several transcriptional factors regulate osteoblast differentiation by regulating Osx.

For instance, knockout mice lacking p53, a well known as tumor suppressor, display a high bone mass phenotype, and p53 knockout osteoblasts show accelerated differentiation, secondary to an increase in expression of Osx, as a result. Reporter assays indicate that p53 represses Osx transcription by the minimal promoter in a DNA-binding-independent manner. Thus p53 suppresses osteoblast differentiation by decreasing Osx levels [67].

MicroRNAs

MicroRNAs (miRNAs) are a class of small molecules and non-coding single strand RNAs with a length of 18-22 nucleotides. They regulate gene expression at the post-transcriptional levels and affect cell growth by regulating processes such as cell proliferation and differentiation [68]. miRNAs can act as both positive and negative factors in the many signaling pathways of the human musculoskeletal system [69]. Studies have shown that miRNAs play an important role in bone biology, such as in osteoblast differentiation and bone formation [70].

There were 22 miRNAs down regulated in the BMP2-induced osteoblast differentiation in a report, suggesting that these miRNAs might inhibit the function of osteoblast differentiation [71].

Activation of FoxO1, the main FoxO in bone, stimulates proliferation and differentiation as well as inhibits apoptosis of osteoblast lineage cells. miR-182 regulates osteoblastogenesis by repressing FoxO1. Over-expression of miR-182 in osteoblast lineage cells increased cell apoptosis and inhibited osteoblast differentiation, whereas in vivo over-expression of miR-182 in zebrafish impaired bone formation. Restoration of FoxO1 expression in miR-182-over-expressed osteoblasts rescued them from the inhibitory effects of miR-182 [72].

In ST2 mouse mesenchymal cells, miR-125b expression is decreased after a 6-day treatment with BMP4. miRNA-125b has a negative effect on osteoblast differentiation, as over-expression of miR-125b decreased ALP activity and knockdown of miR-125b increased the activity of ALP. Potential targets for miR-125b in osteoblasts have not been identified; however, miR-125b may play a role in regulating cell proliferation [73].

miR-133 and miR-135 are down regulated during BMP-2-induced osteoblastic differentiation of C2C12 myoblasts, and in contrast, are up-regulated in these cells during myoblast differentiation [71]. Over-expression of miR-133 or miR-135 blocked the BMP-induced osteoblastic markers, such as ALP, OC, and HOXA10. Further studies demonstrated that Runx2 and Smad5 are targets for miR-133 and Smad5 respectively [74, 75]. The concomitant down-regulation of these two miRNAs by BMP2 likely plays an important role in the up-regulation of Runx2 and Smad5 during osteogenic differentiation.

miR-141 and miR-200a are decreased in BMP2 treated MC3T3-E1 cells. Over-expression of miR-141 and miR-200a decreased protein levels of Dlx5 (Distal-less homeobox 5), which is a critical osteogenic transcriptional factor. In consequence, miR-141 and miR-200a negatively regulated osteoblast differentiation [76, 77].

miR-204 is induced during the adipocyte differentiation of murine C3H10T1/2 cells and human MSCs. Concomitantly, Runx2, a miR-204 target, is decreased. Runx2 is a target for miR-204. Over-expression of miR-204 negatively regulates Runx2 expression, inhibits osteoblast differentiation, and promotes adipocyte differentiation [78].

Runx2 can also be negatively regulated by some members of the miR-23a/27a/24-2 cluster in murine osteoblasts [79].

miR-206 is decreased in response to BMP2 in C2C12 cells and during differentiation of primary murine osteoblasts [80]. Over-expression of miR-206 inhibits ALP activity and Connexin 43 (Cx43). Cx43 is a gap junction protein necessary for osteoblast differentiation and function [81].

Transgenic mice expressing miR-206 in mature osteoblasts display a low bone mass phenotype. Bone formation rate but not osteoclast surface was decreased in miR-206 transgenic mice, suggesting a defect in osteoblast function. These data confirm miR-206 as a negative regulator of osteoblast function.

BMP2 was also shown to decrease the expression of miR-208 [82]. Over-expression of miR-208 antagonized the BMP2-induced osteoblast differentiation of MC3T3-E1 cells and primary mouse osteoblast. The osteogenic transcription factor Ets1 was shown to be a target of miR-208. Ets1 stimulates the transcription of osteopontin and Runx2, and this was inhibited by miR-208 over-expression [82, 83].

During terminal osteoblast differentiation of human adipocyte-derived stem cells, miR-26a increases. Further, as miR-26a increases, Smad1 levels decrease. Smad1 was shown to be a target for miR-26a, and knockdown of miR-26a increased the expression of osteoblast marker genes, including those encoding col1a, osteopontin, and osteocalcin [84].

Prospect for Future Therapy

Osteoporosis, which is one of the most abundant bone related diseases is characterized by low bone mass and microarchitectural deterioration of bone tissue that results in increased bone fragility and susceptibility to fracture [85]. By 2025, the health care expenditures for osteoporotic fractures will approach 25.3 billion dollars [86, 87], highlighting the need for new therapies aimed at preventing the bone loss that normally occurs with aging.

Most commonly prescribed therapeutics are antiresorptives such as calcitonin, estrogen, and bisphosphonates that block osteoclast activity as a means to stabilize bone architecture. While efficacious in halting further bone loss, little or no new bone mass is added to the skeleton while on antiresorptive therapy. Recent data on the importance of continuous bone remodeling as a means to maintain the material and structural strength of bone caution against the overuse of antiresorptives as they may allow for accumulation of microdamage in bone and ultimately lead to fracture in some patients [88]. Thus development of new effective therapies that target enhancing bone formation by stimulating osteoblast offer is required. However such therapies have not spread widely yet.

Enhancing BMP signaling increases bone formation in a variety of animal models, while reducing BMP activity negatively regulates bone mass. Generalized loss of endogenous BMP activity in postnatal mice through over-expression of BMP antagonists by osteoblasts leads to osteopenia, bone fragility and spontaneous fracture [89, 90, 91]. Mice lacking BMP2 are unable to maintain adequate bone formation after birth [9]. BMP in bone declines with age, and this decline correlates with the observation that osteoprogenitors are less effective, replicating, differentiating into osteoblasts and laying down bone matrix in older animals [92, 93, 94]. Short-term systemic administration of BMP2 has been reported to reverse bone loss in osteopenic mice [95]. This effect may be due to rejuvenation of the marrow microenvironment, the niche that harbors osteoprogenitors in adult bone [96]. Additional support for a role for BMP signaling in bone mass regulation comes from studies in which inactivation of BMP3, Tob and CIZ, negative regulators of BMP signaling, lead to increased bone mass in postnatal mice [27, 97, 28, 44, 47]. While these results suggest that activating the BMP-Smad pathway can be beneficial for the skeleton, removal of Bmpr1a, one of the three type I BMP receptors, also leads to enhanced bone formation, most likely by up-regulating Wnt signaling in osteoblasts [98, 99]. This unexpected result suggests that therapeutic approaches aimed at modulating endogenous BMP activity to enhance bone mass will require careful attention to the specific receptor populations present on target cells.

BMPs have been thought to be useful for local bone generation because of their strong bone-inductive effect. Truly BMP2 approved by FDA (Food and Drug Administration) for use in spine fusion surgery in 2002, fracture repair in 2005, and oral and maxillofacial surgery in 2007. However it is difficult to say that clinical application of BMPs has been widespread well because the clinical application of BMPs requires a lot of BMPs and site-specific deliver.

In order to receive the clinical benefit of BMPs we have to identify target cells that BMPs act on to affect to bone regeneration and understand the systems that modulate BMP signaling and osteoblast differentiation followed by. Recently excellent delivery system, which target bone formation surfaces to facilitate RNAi-based anabolic therapy, was reported. This system is involved dioleoyl trimethylammounium propane (DOTAP)-based cationic liposomes attached to six repetitive sequences of aspartate, serine, serine ((AspSerSer)6) for delivering siRNAs specifically to bone formation surfaces [100].

In this chapter BMP signaling and it's regulators, especially inhibitory factors were introduced. Reducing the mRNA expression of these inhibitory factors could be useful for increasing the endogenous BMP signaling. Combination siRNAs against these inhibitors with this delivery system targeting bone formation surfaces may shed light on novel bone formation therapy.

References

[1] Urist, M. R. Bone: formation by autoinduction. *Science* 150, 893-899 (1965).

[2] Urist, M. R. and Strates, B. S. Bone morphogenetic protein. *J. Dent. Res.* 50, 1392-1406 (1971).

[3] Sampath, T. K. and Reddi, A. H. Dissociative extraction and reconstitution of extracellular matrix components involved in local bone differentiation. *Proc. Natl. Acad. Sci. US* 78, 7599-7603 (1981).

[4] Yoshikawa, H., et al. Biochemical stability of a bone-inducing substance from murine osteosarcoma. *Clin. Orthop. Relat. Res.*, 248-253 (1982).

[5] Wozney, J. M., et al. Novel regulators of bone formation: molecular clones and activities. *Science* 242, 1528-1534 (1988).

[6] Sampath, T. K. and Reddi, A. H. Homology of bone-inductive proteins from human, monkey, bovine, and rat extracellular matrix. *Proc. Natl. Acad. Sci. US* 80, 6591-6595 (1983).

[7] Thies, R. S., et al. Recombinant human bone morphogenetic protein-2 induces osteoblastic differentiation in W-20-17 stromal cells. *Endocrinology* 130, 1318-1324 (1992).

[8] Yamaguchi, A., et al. Effects of BMP-2, BMP-4, and BMP-6 on osteoblastic differentiation of bone marrow-derived stromal cell lines, ST2 and MC3T3-G2/PA6. *Biochem. Biophys. Res. Commun.* 220, 366-371, doi:10.1006/bbrc.1996.0411 (1996).

[9] Tsuji, K., et al. BMP2 activity, although dispensable for bone formation, is required for the initiation of fracture healing. *Nat. Genet.* 38, 1424-1429, doi:10.1038/ng1916 (2006).

[10] Katagiri, T., et al. Bone morphogenetic protein-2 converts the differentiation pathway of C2C12 myoblasts into the osteoblast lineage. *J. Cell Biol.* 127, 1755-1766 (1994).

[11] Bianco, P., Robey, P. G., Saggio, I., and Riminucci, M. "Mesenchymal" stem cells in human bone marrow (skeletal stem cells): a critical discussion of their nature, identity, and significance in incurable skeletal disease. *Hum. Gene Ther.* 21, 1057-1066, doi:10.1089/hum.2010.136 (2010).

[12] Wan, M. and Cao, X. BMP signaling in skeletal development. *Biochem. Biophys. Res. Commun.* 328, 651-657 (2005).

[13] Miyazono, K., Maeda, S. and Imamura, T. BMP receptor signaling: transcriptional targets, regulation of signals, and signaling cross-talk. *Cytokine Growth Factor Rev.* 16, 251-263 (2005).

[14] Rosen, V. BMP and BMP inhibitors in bone. *Ann. N Y Acad. Sci.* 1068, 19-25, doi:10.1196/annals.1346.005 (2006).

[15] Katagiri, T., Suda, T. and Miyazono, K. *The bone morphogenetic proteins.* pp-121-149 (Cold Spring Harbor Press, 2008).

[16] Nojima, J., et al. Dual roles of smad proteins in the conversion from myoblasts to osteoblastic cells by bone morphogenetic proteins. *J. Biol. Chem.* 285, 15577-15586, doi:10.1074/jbc.M109.028019 (2010).

[17] Hoodless, P. A., et al. MADR1, a MAD-related protein that functions in BMP2 signaling pathways. *Cell* 85, 489-500 (1996).

[18] Chen, Y., Bhushan, A. and Vale, W. Smad8 mediates the signaling of the ALK-2 [corrected] receptor serine kinase. *Proc. Natl. Acad. Sci. US* 94, 12938-12943 (1997).

[19] Nishimura, R., et al. Smad5 and DPC4 are key molecules in mediating BMP-2-induced osteoblastic differentiation of the pluripotent mesenchymal precursor cell line C2C12. *J. Biol. Chem.* 273, 1872-1879 (1998).

[20] Lopez-Rovira, T., Chalaux, E., Massague, J., Rosa, J. L., and Ventura, F. Direct binding of Smad1 and Smad4 to two distinct motifs mediates bone morphogenetic protein-specific transcriptional activation of Id1 gene. *J. Biol. Chem.* 277, 3176-3185 (2002).

[21] Liu, C. J., Ding, B., Wang, H., and Lengyel, P. The MyoD-inducible p204 protein overcomes the inhibition of myoblast differentiation by Id proteins. *Mol. Cell Biol.* 22, 2893-2905 (2002).

[22] Katagiri, T., et al. Identification of a BMP-responsive element in Id1, the gene for inhibition of myogenesis. *Genes Cells* 7, 949-960 (2002).

[23] Hollnagel, A., Oehlmann, V., Heymer, J., Ruther, U., and Nordheim, A. Id genes are direct targets of bone morphogenetic protein induction in embryonic stem cells. *J. Biol. Chem.* 274, 19838-19845 (1999).

[24] Canalis, E., Economides, A. N. and Gazzerro, E. Bone morphogenetic proteins, their antagonists, and the skeleton. *Endocr. Rev.* 24, 218-235 (2003).

[25] Kameda, T., Koike, C., Saitoh, K., Kuroiwa, A., and Iba, H. Developmental patterning in chondrocytic cultures by morphogenic gradients: BMP induces expression of indian hedgehog and noggin. *Genes Cells* 4, 175-184 (1999).

[26] Pereira, R. C., Economides, A. N. and Canalis, E. Bone morphogenetic proteins induce gremlin, a protein that limits their activity in osteoblasts. *Endocrinology* 141, 4558-4563 (2000).

[27] Daluiski, A., et al. Bone morphogenetic protein-3 is a negative regulator of bone density. *Nat. Genet.* 27, 84-88, doi:10.1038/83810 (2001).

[28] Kokabu, S., et al. BMP3 suppresses osteoblast differentiation of bone marrow stromal cells via interaction with Acvr2b. *Mol. Endocrinol.* 26, 87-94, doi:10.1210/me.2011-1168 (2012).

[29] Gamer, L. W., Cox, K., Carlo, J. M., and Rosen, V. Overexpression of BMP3 in the developing skeleton alters endochondral bone formation resulting in spontaneous rib fractures. *Dev. Dyn.* 238, 2374-2381, doi:10.1002/dvdy.22048 (2009).

[30] Onichtchouk, D., et al. Silencing of TGF-beta signalling by the pseudoreceptor BAMBI. *Nature* 401, 480-485, doi:10.1038/46794 (1999).

[31] Sekiya, T., et al. Identification of BMP and activin membrane-bound inhibitor (BAMBI), an inhibitor of transforming growth factor-beta signaling, as a target of the

beta-catenin pathway in colorectal tumor cells. *J. Biol. Chem.* 279, 6840-6846, doi:10.1074/jbc.M310876200 (2004).

[32] Samad, T. A., et al. DRAGON, a bone morphogenetic protein co-receptor. *J. Biol. Chem.* 280, 14122-14129, doi:10.1074/jbc. M410034200 (2005).

[33] Kanomata, K., Kokabu, S., Nojima, J., Fukuda, T., and Katagiri, T. DRAGON, a GPI-anchored membrane protein, inhibits BMP signaling in C2C12 myoblasts. *Genes Cells* 14, 695-702, doi:10.1111/j.1365-2443.2009.01302.x (2009).

[34] Nakao, A., et al. Identification of Smad7, a TGFbeta-inducible antagonist of TGF-beta signalling. *Nature* 389, 631-635, doi:10.1038/ 39369 (1997).

[35] Imamura, T., et al. Smad6 inhibits signalling by the TGF-beta superfamily. *Nature* 389, 622-626, doi:10.1038/39355 (1997).

[36] Zhu, H., Kavsak, P., Abdollah, S., Wrana, J. L., and Thomsen, G. H. A SMAD ubiquitin ligase targets the BMP pathway and affects embryonic pattern formation. *Nature* 400, 687-693 (1999).

[37] Zhang, Y., Chang, C., Gehling, D. J., Hemmati-Brivanlou, A., and Derynck, R. Regulation of Smad degradation and activity by Smurf2, an E3 ubiquitin ligase. *Proc. Natl. Acad. Sci. US* 98, 974-979, doi:10.1073/pnas.98.3.974 (2001).

[38] Knockaert, M., Sapkota, G., Alarcon, C., Massague, J., and Brivanlou, A. H. Unique players in the BMP pathway: small C-terminal domain phosphatases dephosphorylate Smad1 to attenuate BMP signaling. *Proc Natl. Acad. Sci. US* 103, 11940-11945, doi:0605133103 [pii] 10.1073/ pnas.0605133103 (2006).

[39] Lin, X., et al. PPM1A functions as a Smad phosphatase to terminate TGFbeta signaling. *Cell* 125, 915-928, doi:S0092-8674(06)00517-4 [pii] 10.1016/j.cell.2006.03.044 (2006).

[40] Duan, X., Liang, Y. Y., Feng, X. H., and Lin, X. Protein serine/threonine phosphatase PPM1A dephosphorylates Smad1 in the bone morphogenetic protein signaling pathway. *J. Biol. Chem.* 281, 36526-36532 (2006).

[41] Kokabu, S., et al. Protein phosphatase magnesium-dependent 1A-mediated inhibition of BMP signaling is independent of Smad dephosphorylation. *J. Bone Miner. Res.* 25, 653-660, doi:10.1359/ jbmr.090736 (2010).

[42] Kokabu, S., et al. Suppression of BMP-Smad Signaling Axis-Induced Osteoblastic Differentiation by Small C-terminal Domain Phosphatase 1, a Smad Phosphatase. *Mol. Endocrinol.* 25, 474-481, doi:10.1210/me.2010-0305 (2011).

[43] Ohte, S., et al. Identification and functional analysis of Zranb2 as a novel Smad-binding protein that suppresses BMP signaling. *J. Cell Biochem.* 113, 808-814, doi:10.1002/jcb.23408 (2012).

[44] Yoshida, Y., et al. Negative regulation of BMP/Smad signaling by Tob in osteoblasts. *Cell* 103, 1085-1097 (2000).

[45] Yoshida, Y., et al. Tob proteins enhance inhibitory Smad-receptor interactions to repress BMP signaling. *Mech. Dev.* 120, 629-637 (2003).

[46] Shen, Z. J., et al. Negative regulation of bone morphogenetic protein/Smad signaling by Cas-interacting zinc finger protein in osteoblasts. *J. Biol. Chem.* 277, 29840-29846, doi:10.1074/jbc. M203157200 (2002).

[47] Morinobu, M., et al. The nucleocytoplasmic shuttling protein CIZ reduces adult bone mass by inhibiting bone morphogenetic protein-induced bone formation. *J. Exp. Med.* 201, 961-970, doi:10.1084/ jem.20041097 (2005).

[48] Yukita, A., et al. Ubc9 negatively regulates BMP-mediated osteoblastic differentiation in cultured cells. *Bone* 50, 1092-1099, doi:10.1016/j. bone.2012.02.008 (2012).

[49] Ducy, P., Zhang, R., Geoffroy, V., Ridall, A. L., and Karsenty, G. Osf2/Cbfa1: a transcriptional activator of osteoblast differentiation. *Cell* 89, 747-754, doi:S0092-8674(00)80257-3 [pii] (1997).

[50] Nakashima, K., et al. The novel zinc finger-containing transcription factor osterix is required for osteoblast differentiation and bone formation. *Cell* 108, 17-29, doi:S0092867401006225 [pii] (2002).

[51] Komori, T., et al. Targeted disruption of Cbfa1 results in a complete lack of bone formation owing to maturational arrest of osteoblasts. *Cell* 89, 755-764 (1997).

[52] Otto, F., et al. Cbfa1, a candidate gene for cleidocranial dysplasia syndrome, is essential for osteoblast differentiation and bone development. *Cell* 89, 765-771 (1997).

[53] Mundlos, S., et al. Mutations involving the transcription factor CBFA1 cause cleidocranial dysplasia. *Cell* 89, 773-779 (1997).

[54] Lee, B., et al. Missense mutations abolishing DNA binding of the osteoblast-specific transcription factor OSF2/CBFA1 in cleidocranial dysplasia. *Nat. Genet* .16, 307-310, doi:10.1038/ng0797-307 (1997).

[55] Ducy, P., et al. A Cbfa1-dependent genetic pathway controls bone formation beyond embryonic development. *Genes Dev.* 13, 1025-1036 (1999).

[56] Bialek, P., et al. A twist code determines the onset of osteoblast differentiation. *Developmental cell* 6, 423-435 (2004).

[57] Funato, N., et al. Hand2 controls osteoblast differentiation in the branchial arch by inhibiting DNA binding of Runx2. *Development* 136, 615-625, doi:10.1242/dev.029355 (2009).

[58] Hesse, E., et al. Zfp521 controls bone mass by HDAC3-dependent attenuation of Runx2 activity. *The Journal of cell biology* 191, 1271-1283, doi:10.1083/jcb.201009107 (2010).

[59] Kim, S., et al. Stat1 functions as a cytoplasmic attenuator of Runx2 in the transcriptional program of osteoblast differentiation. *Genes Dev.* 17, 1979-1991, doi:10.1101/gad.1119303 (2003).

[60] Jones, D. C., et al. Regulation of adult bone mass by the zinc finger adapter protein Schnurri-3. *Science* 312, 1223-1227, doi:10.1126/ science.1126313 (2006).

[61] Ohba, S., et al. Patched1 haploinsufficiency increases adult bone mass and modulates Gli3 repressor activity. *Developmental cell* 14, 689-699, doi:10.1016 /j.devcel.2008. 03.007 (2008).

[62] Kanzler, B., Kuschert, S. J., Liu, Y. H., and Mallo, M. Hoxa-2 restricts the chondrogenic domain and inhibits bone formation during development of the branchial area. *Development* 125, 2587-2597 (1998).

[63] Garg, V., et al. Mutations in NOTCH1 cause aortic valve disease. *Nature* 437, 270-274, doi:10.1038/nature03940 (2005).

[64] Hilton, M. J., et al. Notch signaling maintains bone marrow mesenchymal progenitors by suppressing osteoblast differentiation. *Nat. Med.* 14, 306-314, doi:10.1038/nm1716 (2008).

[65] Vega, R. B., et al. Histone deacetylase 4 controls chondrocyte hypertrophy during skeletogenesis. *Cell* 119, 555-566, doi:10.1016/j. cell.2004.10.024 (2004).

[66] Zhou, X., et al. Multiple functions of Osterix are required for bone growth and homeostasis in postnatal mice. *Proc. Natl. Acad. Sci. US* 107, 12919-12924, doi:10.1073/pnas.0912855107 (2010).

[67] Wang, Y., et al. p53 functions as a negative regulator of osteoblastogenesis, osteoblast-dependent osteoclastogenesis, and bone remodeling. *J. Cell. Biol.* 172, 115-125 doi:10.1083/jcb.200507106 (2006).

[68] Bartel, D. P. MicroRNAs: genomics, biogenesis, mechanism, and function. *Cell* 116, 281-297 (2004).

[69] Ambros, V. The functions of animal microRNAs. *Nature* 431, 350-355, doi:10.1038/nature02871 (2004).

[70] Wienholds, E., et al. MicroRNA expression in zebrafish embryonic development. *Science* 309, 310-311, doi:10.1126/science.1114519 (2005).

[71] Li, Z., et al. A microRNA signature for a BMP2-induced osteoblast lineage commitment program. *Proc. Natl. Acad. Sci. US* 105, 13906-13911, doi:10.1073 /pnas.0804438105 (2008).

[72] Kim, K. M., et al. miR-182 is a negative regulator of osteoblast proliferation, differentiation, and skeletogenesis through targeting FoxO1. *J. Bone Miner. Res.* 27, 1669-1679, doi:10.1002/jbmr.1604 (2012).

[73] Mizuno, Y., et al. miR-125b inhibits osteoblastic differentiation by down-regulation of cell proliferation. *Biochem. Biophys. Res. Commun.* 368, 267-272, doi:10.1016/j.bbrc. 2008.01.073 (2008).

[74] Lee, K. S., et al. Runx2 is a common target of transforming growth factor beta1 and bone morphogenetic protein 2, and cooperation between Runx2 and Smad5 induces osteoblast-specific gene expression in the pluripotent mesenchymal precursor cell line C2C12. *Mol. Cell Biol.* 20, 8783-8792 (2000).

[75] Javed, A., et al. Structural coupling of Smad and Runx2 for execution of the BMP2 osteogenic signal. *J. Biol. Chem.* 283, 8412-8422, doi:10.1074/jbc.M705578200 (2008).

[76] Itoh, T., Nozawa, Y. and Akao, Y. MicroRNA-141 and -200a are involved in bone morphogenetic protein-2-induced mouse pre-osteoblast differentiation by targeting distal-less homeobox 5. *J. Biol. Chem.* 284, 19272-19279, doi:10.1074/jbc.M109. 014001 (2009).

[77] Ulsamer, A., et al. BMP-2 induces Osterix expression through up-regulation of Dlx5 and its phosphorylation by p38. *J. Biol. Chem.* 283, 3816-3826, doi:10.1074/jbc. M704724200 (2008).

[78] Huang, J., Zhao, L., Xing, L., and Chen, D. MicroRNA-204 regulates Runx2 protein expression and mesenchymal progenitor cell differentiation. *Stem Cells* 28, 357-364, doi:10.1002/stem.288 (2010).

[79] Hassan, M. Q., et al. A network connecting Runx2, SATB2, and the miR-23a~27a~24-2 cluster regulates the osteoblast differentiation program. *Proc. Natl. Acad. Sci. US* 107, 19879-19884, doi:10.1073/ pnas.1007698107 (2010).

[80] Inose, H., et al. A microRNA regulatory mechanism of osteoblast differentiation. *Proc. Natl. Acad. Sci. US* 106, 20794-20799, doi:10. 1073/pnas.0909311106 (2009).

[81] Lecanda, F., et al. Connexin43 deficiency causes delayed ossification, craniofacial abnormalities, and osteoblast dysfunction. *The Journal of cell biology* 151, 931-944 (2000).

[82] Itoh, T., Takeda, S. and Akao, Y. MicroRNA-208 modulates BMP-2-stimulated mouse preosteoblast differentiation by directly targeting V-ets erythroblastosis virus E26 oncogene homolog 1. *J. Biol. Chem.* 285, 27745-27752, doi:10.1074/jbc.M110.105080 (2010).
[83] Raouf, A. and Seth, A. Ets transcription factors and targets in osteogenesis. *Oncogene* 19, 6455-6463, doi:10.1038/sj.onc.1204037 (2000).
[84] Luzi, E., et al. Osteogenic differentiation of human adipose tissue-derived stem cells is modulated by the miR-26a targeting of the SMAD1 transcription factor. *J. Bone Miner. Res.* 23, 287-295, doi:10.1359/ jbmr.071011 (2008).
[85] Harvey, N., Dennison, E. and Cooper, C. Osteoporosis: impact on health and economics. *Nat. Rev. Rheumatol.* 6, 99-105, doi:10.1038/nrrheum. 2009.260 (2010).
[86] Raisz, L. G. *Overview of patogenesis.* (ASBMR, 2009).
[87] Tosteson, A. *Cost-effectiveness of osteoporosis treatment.* (ASBMR, 2009).
[88] Lenart, B. A., Lorich, D. G. and Lane, J. M. Atypical fractures of the femoral diaphysis in postmenopausal women taking alendronate. *N Engl. J. Med.* 358, 1304-1306, doi:10.1056/NEJMc0707493 (2008).
[89] Gazzerro, E., Gangji, V. and Canalis, E. Bone morphogenetic proteins induce the expression of noggin, which limits their activity in cultured rat osteoblasts. *J. Clin. Invest.* 102, 2106-2114, doi:10.1172/JCI3459 (1998).
[90] Gazzerro, E., et al. Skeletal overexpression of gremlin impairs bone formation and causes osteopenia. *Endocrinology* 146, 655-665, doi:10.1210/en.2004-0766 (2005).
[91] Wu, X. B., et al. Impaired osteoblastic differentiation, reduced bone formation, and severe osteoporosis in noggin-overexpressing mice. *J. Clin. Invest.* 112, 924-934, doi:10.1172/JCI15543 (2003).
[92] Syftestad, G. T. and Urist, M. R. Bone aging. *Clin. Orthop. Relat. Res.*, 288-297 (1982).
[93] Fleet, J. C., Cashman, K., Cox, K., and Rosen, V. The effects of aging on the bone inductive activity of recombinant human bone morphogenetic protein-2. *Endocrinology* 137, 4605-4610 (1996).
[94] Moerman, E. J., Teng, K., Lipschitz, D. A., and Lecka-Czernik, B. Aging activates adipogenic and suppresses osteogenic programs in mesenchymal marrow stroma/stem cells: the role of PPAR-gamma2 transcription factor and TGF-beta/BMP signaling pathways. *Aging Cell* 3, 379-389, doi:10.1111/j.1474-9728.2004.00127.x (2004).
[95] Turgeman, G., et al. Systemically administered rhBMP-2 promotes MSC activity and reverses bone and cartilage loss in osteopenic mice. *J. Cell Biochem.* 86, 461-474, doi:10.1002/jcb.10231 (2002).
[96] Mayack, S. R., Shadrach, J. L., Kim, F. S., and Wagers, A. J. Systemic signals regulate ageing and rejuvenation of blood stem cell niches. *Nature* 463, 495-500, doi:10.1038/nature08749 (2010).
[97] Gamer, L. W., Novc, J., Levin, M., and Rosen, V. BMP-3 is a novel inhibitor of both activin and BMP-4 signaling in Xenopus embryos. *Dev. Biol.* 285, 156-168, doi:10.1016/j.ydbio.2005.06.012 (2005).
[98] Kamiya, N., et al. Wnt inhibitors Dkk1 and Sost are downstream targets of BMP signaling through the type IA receptor (BMPRIA) in osteoblasts. *J. Bone Miner. Res.* 25, 200-210, doi:10.1359/jbmr.090806 (2010).

[99] Kamiya, N., et al. Disruption of BMP signaling in osteoblasts through type IA receptor (BMPRIA) increases bone mass. *J. Bone Miner. Res.* 23, 2007-2017, doi:10.1359/jbmr.080809 (2008).

[100] Zhang, G., et al. A delivery system targeting bone formation surfaces to facilitate RNAi-based anabolic therapy. *Nat. Med.* 18, 307-314, doi: 10.1038/nm.2617 (2012).

In: Osteoblasts
Editor: Hugo Scheurer

ISBN: 978-1-62417-806-1

Chapter 6

The Effect of Molecular and Biochemical Differentiation Agents on Bone Formation

Jafary Farzaneh[1], *Hanachi Parichehr*[2] *and Jafary Fariba*[3]

[1]Faculty of Basic Science, Biology Department, Biochemistry unite, Alzahra University, Tehran, Iran

[2]Faculty of Basic Science, Biology Department, Biochemistry unite, Alzahra University, Tehran, Iran

[3]Departments of Biology, Faculty of Science, Science and Research Branch, IAU, Tehran, Iran

Abstract

This review concisely discusses bone regeneration using cell therapy. Harvesting bone for tissue grafting is a current problem encountered by craniofacial and oral surgeons. Therefore regeneration of fractured or diseased bone is the main subject in tissue engineering. Stem cells derived from human adipose tissue (ADSCs) are multipotent cells that are able to differentiate into osteogenic, chondrogenic and adipogenic lineages and are potential sources for bone production under effect on several agents. The most common supplemental compounds inducing differentiation of stem cells to bone cells in vitro are Ascorbic acid (AA), B-Glycerophosphate (BGP), Dexamethasone (Dex), Bone morphogenic protein 2(BMP-2) Collagen I (col I), and Vetronectin. Information is accommodating on the most important effector that interaction with stem cells and induced differentiation of osteoblast. This present review; try to give a comprehensiveoverview on molecular and biochemical effects of osteoprecursor cells inducers.

Keywords: Bone marker, osteogenic cell, Stem cell, tissue engineering

Introduction

Bone is a major and important organ that plays fundamental and critical roles in human physiology [1]. Bone defectes caused by trauma, cancer, and bone disease (such as osteogenesis imperfect, osteoarthritis, and osteoporosis) highlights the necessity for new procedures and methods in clinical orthopedics. Current treatments are based on different kinds of graft including auto graft, allograft, and xenograft. However these methods are restricted due to pain, donor site morbidity [2-4], paresthesia, risk of deep infection, virus transmition, inflammation, disease transmition, and finally host rejection [5-7]. Thus tissue engineration is considered as an advanced solution for the mentioned problems. The foremost step in bone tissue engineering is the isolation of osteoblast from patient's bone as autologous osteoblast known to be non-immunogenic. These cells have important roles in production and secretion of organic and inorganic bone matrix as well as the control of osteoclast activity. The application of such cells has several limitations including relatively few isolated cells from tissue and low expansion rates of osteoblast. Furthermore in certain bone disease osteoblasts are inappropriate for transplantation [8]. Recently the important role of mesenchymal stem cells in tissue engineering and regeneration has significantly become the focus of attention among researchers [9]. The mesenchymal stem cell is an ideal source because of their ease of access andmultipotency ability to differentiate into osteogenic, chondrogenic and adipogenic lineages [10-12]. Stem cells were first isolated from bone marrow by explantation method [13]. Friedenstein in 1987 reported that bone tissue could be arisen from mesenchymal stem cells [14]. Afterwards,for the first time bone marrow stromal cells was differentiated to osteoblast with osteogenic medium include of dexamethasone, ascorbic acid and glycerol phosphate [15]. Since then many attempts in the differentiation of mesenchymal cells osteoblast was carried out using different inducer. The purpose of this study was to find a way to differentiate the cells faster [16- 21]. The purpose of this study was to review on inducer materials and factors used in the distinction.

Osteoblast Differentiation and Inducer Materials

The cell culture medium is based on the alpha modification of minimal essential medium (a-MEM), supplement with antibiotics, anti-fungal agents, and 15% heat inactivated fetal bovine serum (FBS). According to the original protocol developed by maniatopoulos et al. Some researcher have used complete medium [22] which consists of low-glucose Dulbecco's MEM (DMEM-LG) with 40% fetal bovine serum; while others have used a0MEM as a source of essential nutrients and amino acids [23, 24]. In these cases, serum is chosen to assist cell proliferation however to minimize differentiation, some authors have suggested the addition of different growth factors, either alone or in combination with the complete medium, including epidermal growth factor (EFG), platelet derived growth factor (PDGF) and transforming growth factor B (TGF- B1) , which have been indicated to be strong mitogens for proliferation [23].

Standard Medium for Osteogenic Cultures

The standard culture medium consist of a-MEM 85% $({}^{V}/_{V})$, FBS 15% $({}^{V}/_{V})$ and the following antibiotic-Fungi zone solution: penicillin (167u/ml), gentamicin (50 my/ml) and amphotericin B (0/3my/ml)[22].

Medium Supplements

Additional supplements are added to the standard culture medium so as to promote bone formation in vitro. In original protocol these supplement are dexamethason (Dex 10^{-8}), ascorbic acid (AA, 50mylml), and B- glycerophosphate (B-GP 10mM) [22]. However, modifications in the concentrations of these additions have emerged and would be discussed separately. Recently, researchers have used different supplements for bone engineering as discussed in the following.

Ascorbic Acid

1. The Effect of Ascorobic Acid on Osteoclast Formation

Hagiwara and coworker reported that ascorbic acid might induce the differentiate of osteoclast (ocls) from mouse bone marrow cells and clonal stromal (ST_2) cells. And also they were found that ascorbic acid can induce the formation of tartrate resistant acid phasphatase-positive (TRAP-positive) mononuclear and mul tinucleated cells, which are osteoclast-like cells at concentrations from 0/5 -5 μg/ml. ascorbat act on osteoclast differentiation through the effects on synthesis of RANKL/ODF (receptor activator of NF-κB ligand/osteoclast differentiation factor0 in bone marrow and ST_2 cells [25]. (RANKL/ODF) is a membrane-bound protein that produced by osteoblast / osteogenic stromal cells and have key roles in osteoclastogenesis. It is associetd with the formation of osteoclast-like cells the alloy of osteoclastic precursor cells, and the resorption of bone [26, 27]. Other articles indicated that the impact of 1a,25(OH)2D3 in increasing the level of mRNA for RANKL/ODF is explained elsewhere [27, 28, 29] and it stimulates osteoclastogenesis. Hagiwara reported that association of ascorbic acid and 1a, 25 (OH)2 D3 increased the level of mRNA for RANKL/ODF to 4.7 times in comparision withthe level obtained with 1a,25 (OH)2D3 alone. They suggested that acrobats functions in cooperation with 1a, 25 (OH) 2D3 toward promoting the formation of osteoclast [25].

2.The Effect of Ascorbic Acid on Osteoblast Formation

AA has important roles in intracellular collagene biosynthesis and extracellular calcium deposition in osteoblast and osteoblastic-like cells [30]. AA induced osteoblast differentiation via increased expression of chief genes such as collagen II, Cbfa1/Runx2, Sox , and collagen

X that contribute in both bone mineralization and vascular calcification [31]. Zambuzzi and his colleaguereported that ascorbate could induce osteoblast differentiation through activationof matrix metalloproteinase(MMps) inhibitors such as tissue inhibitors of metalloproteinases (TIMP- 2) and reversion-inducing-cyteine rich protein with kazal motifs(RECK) [32].

Their results provide evidence that RECK and TIMP-2 are involved in the control of ECM remodeling in distinct phases of osteoblast differentiation by modulation MMp activities and a multitude of signaling proteins governs these events [32]. In addition, Farquharson in 1998 indicated that ascorbate enhances 1a,25(OH)2D3 synthesisby upregulation of the vitamin D receptor. He suggested that amplification of the vitamin D receptor is a genomic response against 1a,25(OH)2D3 in elevation of terminal differentiation [32].

Stimulation of the formation of the collagen matrix by AA might be necessary for the formation of ocls. Collagen type I interacts with different type of cells via binding to a_2B_1-integrin [33].

Intraction between collagen and integrin stimulate the osteoblastic differentiation of ST_2 [34] and MC3T3 cells [35, 36], andosteoclast formation as well. Collagen-integrin transduction pathways in mouse preosteoblastic MC3T3 cells induced the binding of Cbfa1 (basic mediator of bone differentiation) to consensus binding site (AACCACT) for Cbfa1 in the 5'-flanking region of the mouse gene for RANKL\ODF [37] without effecting levels of Cbfa1 mRNA [38].

B-Glycerophosphate (BGP)

B-GP is a source of organic phosphate and acts as substrates for alkaline phosphatase (AP). Inorganic phosphate is cleavaged from B-GP with the action of AP [22]. Phosphate is a signal for induction of gene expression and operates as a negative regulator of expression of the osteoblast phosphate transporter gibbon apeleukemia virus receptor [37]. Beck et al reported that osteopontin RNA level is regulated in response to increased extracellular phosphate levels. This protein promotes the attachment of osteoblast and osteoclast to the extracellular matrix [38]. This ability depends on the function of the phosphate transport system.

Furthermore, abundant factors such as B-retinoic acid, endothelin, bone morphogenic protein and vitamin D are known to induce the level of osteopontin in osteoblast and some of these factors induced alkaline phosphatase and increased phosphate levels.

Several studies indicated that high P concentration induce vascular calcification by activated of the Cbfa1/Runx2, the transcription factor core binding factor 1 (Cbfa-1, also called AML-3, Runx-2 and PEBP.2a) is a basic mediator of bone differentiation. Cbfa-1 is desired for osteoblast cell differentiation and regulates the expression of several bone morphogenic proteins [39]. Cozzolino in 2011 was reported that Cbfa1/Runx2 was enhanced under blend stimulate with high P and AA. And also calcium deposition was increased in rat vascular smooth muscle cells (VSMCs) in this condition [40].

Dexamethasone (Dex)

It is currently known that glucocorticoids are potent stimulators of osteoblastic differentiation. Among which, Dexamethasone (a potent synthetic glucocorticoid) is the best according to several studies about its effect on osteoblastic differentiation.

In 2005, Beloti and coworkerstudied the effect of Dex on human BMSC (bone marrow stromal cells). This investigationshowed that continuous and discontinuous Dexs treatment have a positive effect on osteoblast differentiation process. In fact Dex could affect on ALP activity and bone-like formation. Dex at concentrations ranging from 10-7 M to 10-6 M increased the ALP activity. The cells with significant ALP activity also produced mineralized matrix, which indicates a relationship between both markers of osteoblast differentiation [41]. The similar result was reported by Sugawara et al) who revealed that the bone-like formation did not occur in cells without ALP enzymatic activity and its essential for mineralization process of osteoblastic cells [42].

Another study carried out by Katshito et al in 1998, examined the effect of Dex on osteoblastic differentiation in BVSMCs (bovine vascular smooth muscle cells). As shown there, Dex likely promote osteoblastic differentiation of BVSMCs via increasing the expression of the Osf2/Cbfa1 gene. Osf2/Cbfa1 gene is a key regulatory factor in osteoblastic differentiation which recognition recently.

The result emphesized that Dex may induce osteoblastic differentiation of BVSMCs directly and has no effect on their growth [43]. Another studyperformed by Fujita et al showed that Dex induced stimulation of AA uptake by enhanceing expression of Na-dependent vitamin C transporter (SVCT2) mRNA in the mouse osteoblastic cell line. SVCT2 is a gene encoding a transporter with high affinity and specificity for AA. The investigation revealed that there is a glucocorticoids-responsive element in the promoter region of the SVCT2 gene which enhance the gene expression following attachment to the gene [44].

In addition, Dex induced expression of SVCT2 via increasing osteoblastic specific transcription factor. It is a differentiation-associated transcription factor which probably regulate SVCT2 mRNA expression [45].

Vitamin D3

Vitamin D3 metabolites such as 1a, 25-dihydroxy vitamin D3 (1a, 25(OH) 2D3), 25-hydroxy chole calecalciferol (25OH D3) and 19-Nor-1, 25(OH) 2D3 are important regulatory factors in bone metabolism [46-48]. Vitamin D3 metabolites stimulate bone formation though inhibiting the proliferation of osteoblast precursors by induction of the cyclin-dependent kinase inhibitor P21 gene transcription [49, 50]. P21 binds PCNA and blocks PCNA activity [49]. PCNA is a processivity factor for DNA polymerase-σ and key regulator of cell cycle progression [51]. PCNA is increased in the nuclei of cells undergoing mitosis. Slatopolsky et al studied on 19-nor-1, 25(OH) 2D2 and 1, 25(OH) 2D3 and reported that the latter one was more potent on osteoblast proliferation [52].

Vitamin D increased alkaline phosphatase activity and osteocalcin, osteopontin and Gla protein matrix expression [53, 54]. Slatopolsky was indicated that 19-Nor-1, 25(OH) 2D2 and 1, 25(OH) 2D3 were equally potent in increasing of these two markers [52].

Vitamin D metabolites could stimulate the increase of the mRNA levels of the vitamin D receptor (VDR) during osteoblast differentiation [53]. VDR is a member of hormone receptors that act as a transcription factor. This effect by 1, 25(OH) 2 D3 was more than other 19-nor-1, 25(OH) 2D2, 25OH D3 [52, 55].

Bone Morphogenic Protein 2(BMP-2)

Okayama have indicated that BMP-2 induces osteoblast differentiation through binding to the type II receptor and activates the type I receptor leading to formation of R-smad/co-smad complexes, these complexes can express the cdk6 promoter and removing cdk6 exerted blocking of differentiation. The Cdk6 has important roles in determind of the differentiation rate of osteoblast as a downsterm effector of BMP-2/smad signaling [56].

Collagen I and Vetronectin

Collagen I has been shown to induce calcification of stromal cell matrix after 3 weeks [57]. George Ploppr have indicated that Vetronectin (VN) and collagen I (col I) enlarged mineral to matrix ratio, calcium deposition and osteopontin/osteocalcin secretion. Signaling via the col I receptor $\alpha_1\beta_1$ integrin and the VN receptor $\alpha v\beta_3$ integrin plays the most important role in prompting osteogenesis. In summary their results have shown that at least two different extra cellular matrix proteins (Vetronectin, collagen I) and their corresponding integrin receptors, prompt osteogenic differentiation without soluble osteogenesis factors, and may control integrin signaling pathway in human mesenchymal stromal stem cells differentiation [58].

Conclusion and Further Remarks

A variety of materials have been used for differentiation of stem cells into osteogenic cells. Most of which induce bone formations via increasing the levels of bone markers. The research in the field of bone tissue regeneration is under way. New inducers with higher osteogenic capability would prospectively being discovered. A substantial part of this review is committed to the molecular and chemical mechanism of inducing materials that will help researchers to use supplement medium with greatest effect on osreogenic differentiation.

References

[1] AAOS. http://www. Aaos.org/research/patientstats. [20 August 2008] American academy of orthopedic surgeons.

[2] Silber JS, Anderson DG, Daffner SD, Brislin BT, Leland JM,Hilibrand AS. Donor site morbidity after anteriSilbor iliac crest bone harvest for single-level anterior cervical discectomy and fusion. *Spine,* 2003; 28: 134–139.

[3] Arrington ED, Smith WJ, Chambers HG, Bucknell AL, DavinoNA. Complications of iliac crest bone graft harvesting. *Clin. Orthop. Relat. Res.,* 1996; 329: 300–309.

[4] Banwart JC, Asher MA, Hassanein RS. Iliac crest bone graft harvest donor site morbidity. *A statistical evaluation. Spine,* 1995; 20:1055–1060.

[5] Mankin HJ, Hornicek FJ, Raskin KA. Infection in massive bone allografts. *Clin. Orthop. Relat. Res.,* 2005; 432: 210–216.

[6] Lanza RP, Butler DH, Borland KM, Staruk JE, Faustman DL,Solomon BA et al. Xenotransplantation of canine, bovine, and porcine isletsin diabetic rats without immunosuppression. *Proc. Natl. Acad. Sci. USA,* 1991; 88:11100–11104.

[7] Yoo D, Giulivi A. Xenotransplantation and the potential risk of xenogeneic transmission of porcine viruses. *Can. J. Vet. Res.,* 2000; 64:193–203.

[8] Heath CA. Cells for tissue engineering. *Trends Biotech* 2000; 18: 17-18.

[9] Caplan AI, Bruder SP. Mesenchymal stem cells: building blocks for molecular medicine in the 21st century. *Trends Mol. Med.,* 2001; 7:259-264.

[10] Baksh D, song L, Tuan RS. Adult Mesenchymal stem cells: characterization differentiation, and application in cell and gene therapy. *J. Cell Mol. Med.,* 2004; 8:301-316.

[11] Pittenger MF, Mackay AM, Beck SC, Jaiswal RK, Douglas R, Mosca JD. Multilineage potential of adult human Mesenchymal stem cells. *Science,* 1999; 284: 143-147.

[12] Prockop DJ. Marrow stromal cells as stem cells for nanhematopoietic tissue. *Science,* 1997; 276:71-74.

[13] Friedenstein AJ, Gorskaja UF, Kulagina NN. Fibroblast precursors in normal and irradiated mouse hematopoietic organs. *Exp. Hematol.,* 1976; 4: 267-74.

[14] Friedenstein AJ, Chailakhyan RK, Gerasimov UV. Bone marrow osteogenic stem cells: In vitro cultivation and transplantation in diffusion chambers. *Cell Proliferat.,* 1987; 20: 263-72.

[15] Maniatipoulos C, sodek J, Melcher AH. Bone formation in vitro by stromal cells obtained from bone marrow of young adult rats. *Cell Tissue Res.,* 1988; 254: 317-30.

[16] Liu P, Oyajobi Bo, Russell RGG, Scutt A. Regulation of osteogenic differentiation of human bone marrow stromal cells: interaction between transforming growth factor- B and b25 (OH) 2 vitamin D3 in vitro. *Calcif. Tissue Int.,* 1999; 65: 173-800.

[17] Jain RK, Vuorinen A, Sandor GKB, Suuronen R, Miettinen S. Vitamin D_3 metabolites induce osteogenic differentiation in human dental pulp and human dental follicle cells. *Journal of steroid Biochemistry and Molecular Biology,* 2010; 122: 133-41.

[18] Colter DC, Class R, Digirolamo CM, Prockop DJ. Rapid expansion of recycling stem cells cultures of plastic-adherent cells from human bone marrow. *Proc. Natl. Acad. Sci.,* 2000; 97: 3213-3218.

[19] Pittenger MF, Mackay AM, Beak SC, Jaiswal RK, Douglas R, Mosca JD, Moorman MA, Craig S, Marshak DR. Multilineage potential of adult human mesenchymal stem cells. *Science,* 1999; 248: 141-147.

[20] Mendes SC, Bruijn JD, Bakker K, Apeldoorn A, Platenburg P, Tibbe G. J. M, Van Blitt swijk CA. Human bone marrow stromal cells for bone-tissue engineering: In vitro and in vivo characterition. *Bone Engineering,* 2000; 47: 505-515.

[21] Phinney DG, Kopen G, Isaacsson RL, Prockop DJ. Plastic adherent stromal cells from the bone marrow of commonly used strains of inbred mice: Variations in yield, growth, and differentiation. *J. Cell Physiol.,* 1999; 91: 335-344.

[22] Atala A, Lanza R .2002. Methods of Tissue engineering. In: Davies J, Karp M, Baksh D (ed) Mesenchymal cell culture: Bone, firth end. Academic press: pp; 333-345.

[23] Otsuka E, Kato Y, Hirose S, Hagiwara H. Role of ascorbic acid in the osteoclast formation: induction of osteoclast differentiation factor with formation of extracellular collagen matrix. *Endocrinology,* 2000; 141: 306-311.

[24] Lacey DL, Timms E, Tan HL, Kelley MJ, Dunstan CR, Burgess T et al. Osteoprotegerin ligand is a cytokine that regulates osteoclast differentiation and activation. *Cell,* 1998; 93: 165-176.

[25] Yasuda H, Shima N, Nakagawa N, Yamaguchi K, Kinosaki M, Mochizuki S et al. Osteoclast differentiation factor is a ligand for osteoprotegerin /osteoclastogenesis – inhibitory factor and identical to TRANCE/RANkl. *Proc. Natl. Acad. Sci.,* 1998; 95; 3597-3602.

[26] Tsukii K, Shima N, Mochizuki S, Yamaguchi K, Kinosaki M, Yano K. Osteoclast differentiation factor mediates an essential signal for bone resorption induced by 1a, 25-Dihidroxyvitamin D3 prostaglandin E_2 or patathyroid hormone in the microenviroment or bone. *Biochem. Biophys. Res. Commun.,* 1998; 246: 337-341.

[27] Horwood NJ, Elliott J, Martin TJ, Gillespie MT. Osteotropic agents regulate the expression of osteoclast differentiation factor and osteoprotegerin in osteoblast stromal cells. *Endocrinology,* 1998; 139: 4743-4746.

[28] Farquharson C, Berry JL, Mawer EB. Ascorbic acid-induced chondrocytes terminal differentiation: the role of extracellular matrix and 1,25-dihydroxyvitamin D. *Eur. J. Cell Biol.,* 1998; 76: 110-118.

[29] Altaf FM, Hering TM, Kazmi NH. Ascorbate-enhanced chondrogenesis of At DC5 cells. *Eur. Cell Mater.,* 2006; 12: 64-69.

[30] Willian F, Zambuzzi L, Alexander DM, Cavagis P, Granjeiro JM, Carmen V. Ascorbate-induced osteoblast differentiation recruits distinct MMP-inhibitors: RECK and TIMP-2. *Mol. Cell Biochem.,* 2008; 322: 143-150.

[31] Clark EA, Brugge Js. Integrins and signal transduction oathways: the road taken. *Science,* 1995; 268: 233-239.

[32] Otsuka E, Yamaguchi A, Hirose S, Hagiwara H. Characterization of osteoblastic differentiation of stromal cell line ST2 that is induced by ascorbic acid. *Am. J. Physiol.,* 1999; 277: 132-138.

[33] Takeuchi Y, Nakayama K, Matsumoto T. Differentiation and cell surface expression of transforming growth factor-B receptors are regulated by interaction with matrix collagen in murine osteoblastic cells. *J. Biol. Chem.,* 1996; 271: 3938-3944.

[34] Takeuchi Y, Suzawa M, Kikuchi T, Nishida E, Fujita T, Matsumoto T. Differentiation and transforming growth factor-B receptor down-regulation by collagen –a2B1 integrin intraction is mediated by focal adhesion kinase and its downstream signals in murine osteoblastic cells. *J. Biol. Chem.,* 1997; 272: 29309-29316.

[35] Kitazawa R, Kitazawa S, Maeda S. Promotor structure of mouse RANKL/TRANCE/OPGL/ODF gene. *Biochim. Biophys. Acta,* 1999; 1445:134-141.

[36] Xiao G, Wang D, Benson MD, Karsenty G, Franceschi RT. Role of the a2-integrin in osteoblast-specific gene expression and activation of the Osf2 transcription factor. *J. Biol. Chem.*, 1998; 273: 32988-3299.

[37] Kavanaugh MP, Miller DG, Zhang W, Law W, Kozak S, Kabat D, Miler D. Cell-surface receptors for gibbon ape leukemia virus and amphotropic murine retrovirus are inducible sodium-dependent phosphate symporters. *Proc. Natl. Acad. Sci.*, 1994; 91: 7071-7075.

[38] George R, Beck Jr, Brad Zerler, Moran E. Phosphat is a specific signal for induction of osteopontin gene expression. *PNAS*, 2000; 97: 8352-8357.

[39] Zaragoza C, López-Rivera E, García-Rama C, Saura M, Martínez-Ruíz A, Lizarbe T, Martín-de-Lara F, Lamas S. Cbfa-1 mediates nitric oxide regulation of MMP-13 in osteoblasts. *J. of Cell Science*, 2006; 119: 1896-1902.

[40] Ciceri P, Volpi E, Brenna I, Arnaboldi L, Neri L, Brancaccio D. Combined effects of ascorbic acid and phosphate on rat VSMC osteoblastic differentiation. *Nephrol. Dial. Transplant.*, 2012; 27: 122-127.

[41] Ettore L, Francesca M, Silvia CS, Isabella T, Gianna G, Maria LB. Osteogenic Differentiation of Human Adipose Tissue–Derived Stem Cells Is Modulated by the miR-26a Targeting of the SMAD1 Transcription Factor. *J. bone mine. Res*., 2008; 23:287-295.

[42] Sugawara Y, Suzuki K, Koshikawa M,Ando M,Iida j. necessity of enzymatic activity of alkaline phosphatase for minarization of osteoblastic cells. *Jpn. J. pharmacol.*, 2002; 88:262-269.

[43] Katsuhito M, Atsushi S, Shuichi J, Yoshiki N ,Hirotoshi M. Dexamethasone Enhances In Vitro Vascular Calcification by Promoting Osteoblastic Differentiation of Vascular Smooth Muscle Cells. *J. Am. heart associate,* 1999; 19:2112-2118.

[44] Fujita I, Hirano J, Itoh N, Nakanishi T , Tanaka K. Dexamethasone induces sodium-dependant vitamin C transporter in a mouse osteoblastic cell line MC3T3-E1. *British J. Nutrition,* 2001; 86:145–149.

[45] Chang DJ , Ji C, Kim KK, Casinghino S, McCarthy TL, Centrella M. reduction in transforming growth factor beta receptor I experisson and transcription factor CBFα1 on bone cells by glucocorticoid . *J. biological chem.*, 1998; 173: 4892-4896.

[46] Van Driel M, Pols HA, Leeuwen JP. Osteoblast differentiation and control by vitamin D and vitamin D metabolites. *Curr. Pharm. Des.*, 2004; 10: 2535-2555.

[47] Christakos S, Dhawan P, Liu X, Porta A. New insights in to the mechanism of vitamin D action. *J. Cell Biochem.*, 2003; 88: 695-705.

[48] Jean G, Terrat JC, Vanel T, Hurot JM, Lorriaux C, Mayor B, Chazot C. Daily oral 25-hydroxycholecaliferol supplement for vitamin D deficiency in haemodialysis patient: effect on mineral metabolism and bone markers. *Dial. Transplant.*, 2008; 23:3670-3676.

[49] Waga S, Hannon GJ, Beach D, Sullivan B. The P21 inhibitor of cyclin-dependent kinase controls DNA replication by interaction with PCNA. *Nature,* 1994; 369: 574-578.

[50] Liu M, Lee MH, Cohen M, Bommakanti M, Freedman LP. Transcriptional activation of the Cdk inhibitor P21 by vitamin D3 leads to the induced differentiation of myelomonocytic cell line U937. *Genes Dev.*, 1996; 10:142-153.

[51] Almendral JM, Huebsch D, Blundell PA, Macadonald-Bravo H, Bravo R. Cloning and sequence of the human nuclear protein cyclin: Homology with DNA-binding proteins. *Proc. Natl. Acad. Sci. USA,* 1987; 84: 1575-1987.

[52] Jane L, Adriana S, Tricia P, Eduardo A. Relation potencies of 1,25(OH)2D3 and 19-Nor-1,25(OH)2D2 on inducing differentiation and markers of bone formation in MG-63 cells. *J. Am. Soc. Nephrol.,* 2001; 12:1468-1474.

[53] Van Driel, Koedam M, Buurman CJ, Roelse M, Weyts F, Chiba AG. Evidence that both 1alpha,25-dihydroxyvitamin D3 and 24-hydroxyvitamin D3benhance human osteoblast differentiation and mineralization. *J. Cell Biochem.,* 2008; 99: 922-935.

[54] Shiba H, Uchida Y, Kamihagi K, Sakate M, Fujita T, Nakamura S. Transforming growth factor-beta1 and basic fibroblast growth factor modulate osteocalcin and osteonectin/SPARC syntheses in vitamin-D-activated pulp cells. *J. Dent. Res.,* 2001; 80:1653-1659.

[55] Jain R, Vuorinen A, Sandor G, Suuronen R, miettinen S. Vtamin D3 metabolites induce osteogenic differentiation in human dental pulp and human dental follicle cells. *J. Steroid. Biochem. Molecular Biology,* 2010; 122:133-141.

[56] Ogasawara T, Kawaguchi H, Jinno S, Hoshi K, Itaka K, Takato T. Bone morphogenetic protein 2-induced osteoblast differentiation requires smad-mediated down-regulation of Cdk6. *Molecular Cell Biology,* 2004; 24: 6560-6568.

[57] Mizuno M, Kuboki Y. Osteoblast-related gene expression of bone marrow cells during the osteoblastic differentiation induced by type I collagen. *J. Biochem.,* 2001; 129:133-138.

[58] Salasznyk R, Williams W, Boskey A, Batorsky A, Plopper G. Adhesion to vitronectin and collagen I promote osteogenic differentiation of human mesenchymal stem cells. *J. Biomed. Biotechnol.,* 2003; 1: 24-34.

In: Osteoblasts
Editor: Hugo Scheurer

ISBN: 978-1-62417-806-1

Chapter 7

Evaluation of Characteristics of Osteoblasts and Factors Related to Osteoblastic Differentiation and Mineralization

Jun-Beom Park*
Department of Periodontics, Seoul St Mary's Hospital,
College of Medicine, The Catholic University of Korea,
Seoul, Korea

Abstract

Osteoblasts play a key role in bone formation and it expresses bone-related protein such as bone sialoprotein and osteocalcin. The morphology of osteoblast may change related to the environment. The attachment, proliferation and differentiation depend on the local and systemic condition.

There are so many diseases that are related to the function of osteoblasts. It is widely accepted that estrogen deficiency may be the principal cause of postmenopausal osteoporosis, and that the direct effects of estrogen on bone-forming osteoblasts is very important in the progression of the disease.

In this review, the change of the osteoblasts depending on the surrounding environment is describd. Moreover, the change of function and clinical implications will be extensively reviewed.

Keywords: Osteoblast, bone, morphology, function, attachment, proliferation, differentiation, estrogen

---

* Corresponding Author: Jun-Beom Park DDS, MSD, PhD. Department of Periodontics, Seoul St Mary's Hospital, College of Medicine, The Catholic University of Korea, 222, Banpo-daero, Seocho-gu, Seoul 137-701, Republic of Korea, Phone: +1-82-18-325-2651, E-mail: jbassoonis@yahoo.co.kr.

Introduction

Osteoblasts are reported to play a key role in bone formation. The morphology of osteoblast may change related to the environment [1]. The attachment, proliferation and differentiation depend on the local and systemic condition [2-4]. There are so many diseases that are related to the function of osteoblasts [5, 6]. It is widely accepted that estrogen deficiency may be the principal cause of postmenopausal osteoporosis, and that the direct effects of estrogen on bone-forming osteoblasts is very important in the progression of the disease [7]. In this report, the change of the osteoblasts depending on the surrounding environment is describd. Moreover, the change of function and clinical implications will be extensively reviewed.

Characteristics of Osteblast

Osteoblasts are mesenchymal origin cells responsible for creating and maintaining skeletal architecture [8]. These pluripotent mesenchymal stem cells are reported to have the capability to be differentiated into bone, cartilage and adipose tissue, depending on the activated signaling transcription pathways [9, 10]. Osteoblasts are considered mononucleate cells and they have morphologic charisteristics of fibroblast (Figure 1).

Core-binding factor α1 (Cbfa1), belonging to the runt-domain gene family is reported to be an osteoblast-specific transcription factor [11]. It is known to be responsible for the commitment of pluripotent mesenchymal cells into the osteoblast cell lineage.and it serves as a regulator of osteoblast differentiation [8, 12].

Osteoblast commitment, growth and differentiation are modulated by several local and systemic factors [8] (Figure 2). A wide ragen of cytokines growth factors are involved in regulating osteoblast differentiation and function [13].

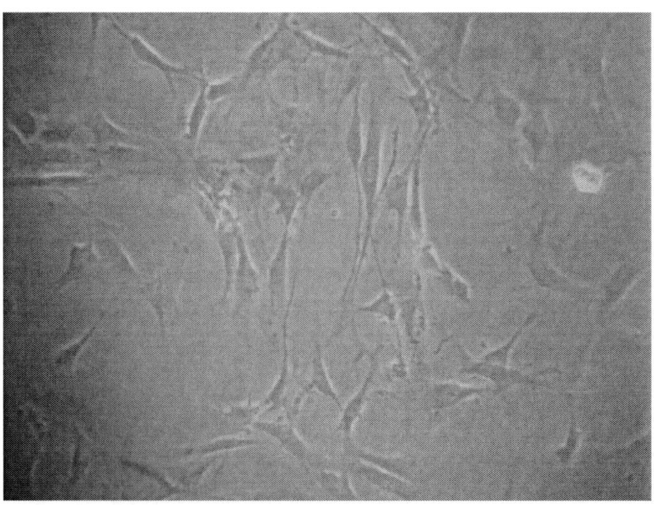

Figure 1. Morphology of the osteoblast-like cells under a light microscope.

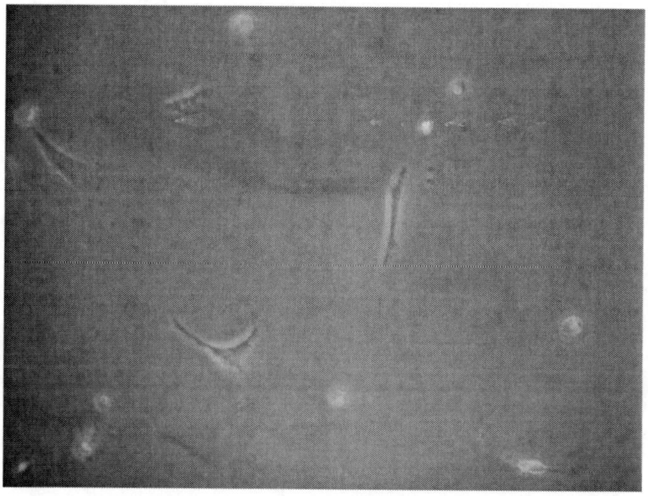

Figure 2. Change of morphology of the osteoblast-like cells due to the local factor.

It was suggested that primary molecular agents may induce secondary responses by the target cells, influencing, in turn, the cellular dynamics of bone in an autocrine or paracrine manner [13]. Expression of osteocalcin synthesis is reported to occur subsequent to initiation of alkaline phosphatase activity and accompanies the formation of mineralized nodules in cultured osteoblasts [14]. During the osteoblastic differentiation, the formation of collagen cross-links (pyridinoline and deoxypyridinoline) was time-dependently accelerated with the accumulation of collagens and this coincided with an onset of mineralization of the cultures [15]. mRNA expression of bone morphogenetic proteins (BMPs) revealed a notable elevation [15]. Growth factors including BMP, platelet-derived growth factor, basic fibroblast growth factor, and transforming growth factor-β are reported to be involved in osteoblast differentiation. There has been considerable interest in their use as therapeutic agents in the treatment of bone disorders, as growth factors become available as therapeutic agents with the advent of recombinant growth factor [13].

Bone Morphogenetic Protein (BMP)

Attempts have been made to promote the bone formation using growth factors, such as bone morphogenetic proteins (BMPs) [16, 17]. BMPs are members of the transforming growth factor-β superfamily and have been known to induce heterotopic bone formation [18]. BMPs are reported to have osteoinductive properties, and favorable regenerative responses to the graft materials containing BMPs have been reported [17]. BMP-2 is reported to induce alkaline phosphatase expression and extracellular matrix mineralization by osteoblasts [19]. The BMP and Wnt/β-catenin signaling pathways cooperatively regulate osteoblast differentiation and bone formation, and it is known that BMP signaling regulates gene expression of the Wnt pathway [5].

Various Agents

Simvastatin is a chemical modification of lovastatin, a rate-limiting enzyme of the cholesterol synthesis pathway [20]. Simvastatin has been demonstrated to promote osteoblastic activity [21]. Simvastatin promoted differentiation by partially regulating the expressions of ER-α, while maintaining osteoblastic viability [22]. The combination of simvastatin and BMP-2 produced positive effects on the differentiation of osteoprecursor cells and the results also suggest that the combination of simvastatin and BMP-2 has synergistic effects that are achieved through the BMP pathway by enhancing the expression of pSmad1/5/8 expression [23].

Laboratory Experiments

The effect on cell viability is determined by 3-[4,5-dimethylthiazol-2-yl]-2,5-diphenyltetrazolium bromide (MTT) assay [23]. Osteoblastic differentiation and mineralization are examined using an alkaline phosphatase activity test and alizarin red-S staining, respectively [24].

(1) Cellular Proliferation

Cells are loaded in culture plate or multi-well and cells are challenged with different dosage of multiple agents. At the end of the incubation time, the MTT reagents are added with final concentration of 0.5 mg/mL. The cells are then incubated for 1 to 4 h at 37°C depending on the condition. Washing with phosphate-buffered saline (PBS, pH 7.4) is followed by the addition of DMSO.

Complete dissolution can be achieved after gentle shaking. Aliquots of the resulting solutions are transferred in 96-well plates, and absorbance is recorded at 560 nm and 670 nm using the microplate spectrophotometer system (Figure 3).

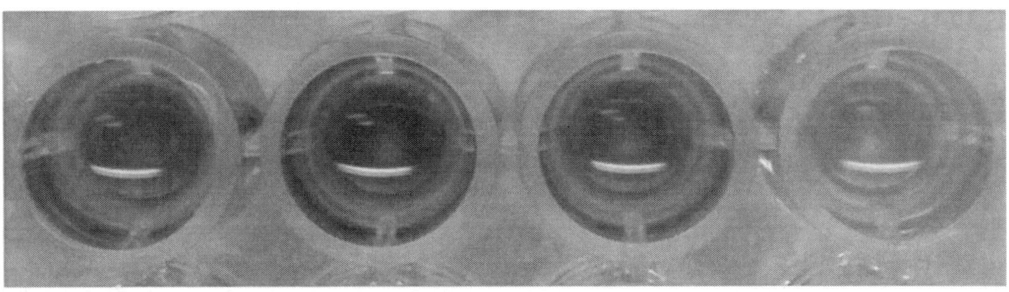

Figure 3. Determination of cellular proliferation using the MTT assay.

(2) Alkaline Phosphatase Activity Assays (ALP)

Cells are lysed into buffer containing 10 mM Tris–HCl pH 7.4, 0.2 % Triton X-100 and then sonicated at 4°C. Samples are added to glycine buffer (100mM, pH 10.5) containing 10 mM p-nitrophenylphosphate and 1mM $MgCl_2$ and incubated at 37°C in a water bath. Total protein content is determined in comparison with series of bovine albumin serum as internal standards. The optical density of p-nitrophenol at 405 nm is determined spectrophotometrically (Figure 4). ALP activities are normalized with respect to total protein content.

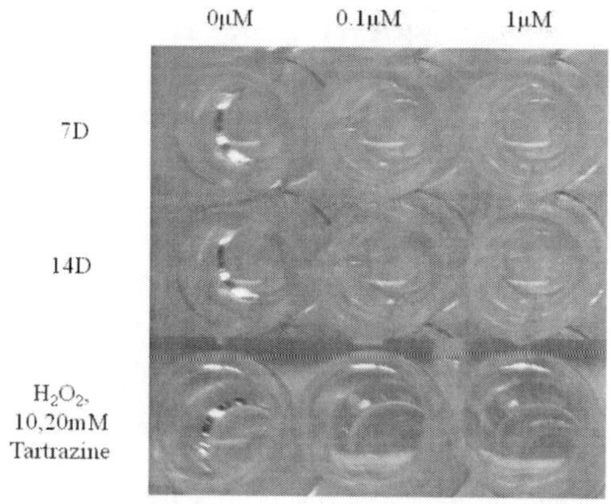

Figure 4. Evaluation of ALP activity.

(3) Mineralization Assay

Cell cultures obtained are washed twice with phosphate-buffered saline, fixed for 1 h in ice-cold 70% ethanol, and rinse twice with deionized water. The cultures are stained with 40 mM alizarin red S for 30 min under gentle shaking. To remove non-specifically bound stain, cultures are washed three times with deionized water and once with PBS for 15 minutes at an ambient temperature (Figure 5). To quantify the bound dye, the stain is solubilized with 10% cetyl pyridinium chloride by shaking. The absorbance of the solubilized stain is measured at 562 nm.

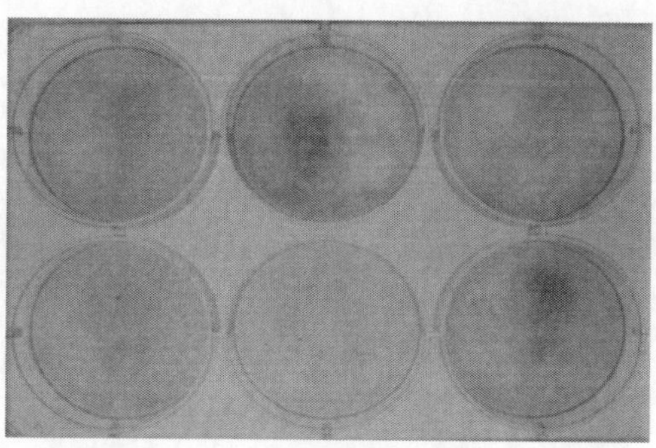

Figure 5. Evaluation of mineralization after staining with alizarin red-S solution.

Conclusion

In this paper, the effect of local and systemic condition on the osteoblastic differentiation is described. Moreover, laboratory techniques regarding the evaluation of the cellular proliferation, differentiation and mineralization are reviewed. Further studies using *in vitro* and *in vivo* models are needed to evaluate the relationship between local and systemic factors and osteoblastic differentiation.

References

[1] A. Hoebertz, S. Mahendran, G. Burnstock and T. R. Arnett, *J. Cell Biochem.* 86, 413 (2002).

[2] A. S. Weaver, Y. P. Su, D. L. Begun, J. D. Miller, A. I. Alford and S. A. Goldstein, *Bone.* 47, 41 (2010).

[3] A. Ponche, M. Bigerelle and K. Anselme, *Proc. Inst. Mech. Eng. H.* 224, 1471 (2010).

[4] K. Anselme, A. Ponche and M. Bigerelle, *Proc. Inst. Mech. Eng. H.* 224, 1487 (2010).

[5] R. Zhang, B. O. Oyajobi, S. Harris, *et al.*, *Bone.* (2012).

[6] R. Tabrizi, A. M. Arabi, H. R. Arabion and M. Gholami, *J. Craniofac. Surg.* 21, 136 (2010).

[7] K. M. Waters, D. J. Rickard, B. L. Riggs, *et al.*, *J. Cell Biochem.* 83, 448 (2001).

[8] A. Neve, A. Corrado and F. P. Cantatore, *Cell Tissue Res.* 343, 289 (2011).

[9] T. L. Arinzeh, S. J. Peter, M. P. Archambault, *et al.*, *J. Bone Joint Surg. Am.* 85-A, 1927 (2003).

[10] J. B. Park, S. S. Bae, P. W. Lee, *et al.*, *Tissue Eng. Regen Med.* 9, 224 (2012).

[11] P. Ducy, R. Zhang, V. Geoffroy, A. L. Ridall and G. Karsenty, *Cell.* 89, 747 (1997).

[12] Z. S. Xiao, T. K. Hinson and L. D. Quarles, *J. Cell Biochem.* 74, 596 (1999).

[13] F. J. Hughes, W. Turner, G. Belibasakis and G. Martuscelli, *Periodontol. 2000.* 41, 48 (2006).

[14] M. A. Aronow, L. C. Gerstenfeld, T. A. Owen, M. S. Tassinari, G. S. Stein and J. B. Lian, *J. Cell Physiol.* 143, 213 (1990).

[15] N. Yamamoto, K. Furuya and K. Hanada, *Biol. Pharm Bull.* 25, 509 (2002).

[16] P. J. Boyne, L. C. Lilly, R. E. Marx, *et al.*, *J. Oral Maxillofac. Surg.* 63, 1693 (2005).

[17] J. B. Park, *J. Craniofac Surg.* 20, 1501 (2009).

[18] J. B. Park, J. Y. Lee, H. N. Park, *et al.*, *J Periodontol.* 78, 157 (2007).

[19] G. Rawadi, B. Vayssiere, F. Dunn, R. Baron and S. Roman-Roman, *J. Bone Miner Res.* 18, 1842 (2003).

[20] J. B. Park, *Med Oral Patol Oral Cir Bucal.* 14, e485 (2009).

[21] K. H. Baek, W. Y. Lee, K. W. Oh, *et al.*, *J. Korean Med. Sci.* 20, 438 (2005).

[22] J. B. Park, H. Zhang, C. Y. Lin, *et al.*, *J. Surg. Res.* (2011).

[23] J. B. Park, *Exp. Ther. Med.* 4, 303 (2012).

[24] J. B. Park, *Exp. Ther. Med.* 4, 681 (2012).

Index

C

D

E

F

G

H

I

J

K

L

N

O

P

Q

R

S

T

U

V

W

Y

Z